THE MEN'S CLUB

HOW TO LOSE YOUR PROSTATE WITHOUT LOSING YOUR SENSE OF HUMOR

"The Men's Club"*

How to Lose Your Prostate Without Losing Your Sense of Humor

by
Bert Gottlieb, patient
Thomas Mawn, M.D.

*Where women are always welcome.

THE MEN'S CLUB

Published By
Pathfinder Publishing
3600 Harbor Boulevard, # 82
Oxnard, CA 93035, U.S.A.

Copyright 1999 by Bert Gottlieb, and Thomas Mawn

First Printing 1999

Library of Congress Cataloging-in-Publication Data

Gottlieb, (Bert), 1999
    The Men's Club: How To Lose Your Prostate without
losing Your Sence of Humor / by Bert Gottlieb, and Thomas Mawn
MD
    p. cm
Includes bibliographical references
ISBN 0-934793-67-0
    1. Health & Medical

PREFACE

This book is the history of a diseased prostate, chronicled by both patient and doctor from discovery through removal to survival.

The reason for both points of view is because there are two sides to every prostate: the side the doctor can initially touch and snip tissue from, and the side that's out of reach, yet irrevocably part of the patient. So it is with prostate cancer: the doctor on one side of the fray, his patient on the other. For the whole picture you need both sides.

And while this is a record of but one prostate's progress, as of today, many men will likely share the same experiences once they hear the words "You have prostate cancer."

Of course, by the time this account will have appeared in print, newer techniques in surgery and radiotherapy, more specific testing procedures, even finer analyses and hopefully, better answers to the thorny questions having prostate cancer raises, will no doubt have come about and will continue to develop. But barring a paradigm shift in medical technology, the steps taken, and the difficult trek toward a patient's survival, will basically remain the same as described herein.

If this chronicle imparts any insights into the process of surviving prostate cancer, great. If it provides some hope, even better.

Bert Gottlieb & Thomas Mawn

Acknowledgements

We would like to thank our respective families, friends, and business and professional associates for their incredible encouragement while this book was being born, with special thanks to Nancy Frederich who fly-specked the original manuscript, making many important catches; and Dr. James Biemer, former Chairman of the Department of Pathology at St. Joseph's Hospital in Tampa, for going over the book after recovering from prostate surgery himself. And our enduring gratitude to the book's biggest fan and toughest critic: Rose.

CONTENTS

Introduction

From the day a man is born, he is automatically enrolled in The Men's Club, most obviously because he was lucky enough to be born a man, and like every man, unlucky enough to have a prostate.

Some men have breasts. Other men, if they're willing to undergo a sex change, can have a sort of vagina; so too, can a woman have a sort of penis. But when it come to plumbing, a woman can't have a prostate, just like a man can't have ovaries or a uterus. That's just the way things are, Professor 'Iggins. Politically incorrect, perhaps, but glands do tend to be apolitical.

Of course, if a woman has a man she cares about, she's automatically welcome to the Club. Once inside, she can listen to all the tales of prostates gone awry, all the dirty talk of unspoken fears, and more important, learn enough about prostate cancer to make sure her man isn't kicked out of the club before his time, since men don't talk about their private lives the way women do. Women are savvy enough to share important stuff about important, albeit private, matters.

About as private as a man usually gets is to boast about his privates. Impotency is treated as a joke. *What's the matter, Vinny—can't get it up?* But tell another guy he can't get it up? Or that he has to wear a diaper because of incontinence? Too un-macho. *I can't admit there's something wrong down there.* The guys'd laugh at me! Like Richard Pryor, they can only grab their crotches and make dick jokes. And when the situation isn't funny anymore, they clam up, allowing the sadness to destroy their insides as surely as their prostate cancer will. They'll ignore their dirty little secret and its symptoms and never question the cause, even if it winds up killing them.

With even the mildest BPH symptoms, you'll rarely hear a man announce to his pals, "Gee, it's taking me so long to start peeing."

Or: "Seems like I'm always having to whiz." That would be an admission of serious aging, of the loss of some unverbalized, primal force that can never be admitted to, even when there's no denying the facts; it would be cause for a joke. The hardest thing about being a man, it seems, is admitting to it.

Which is why women are always welcome to The Men's Club. It desperately needs their openness and their ability to face unfunny truths squarely, their understanding of the fact that one loss doesn't count for everything, and that there's nothing shameful or humorous when it comes to medical problems.

Without women, The Men's Club is a joke. So please, ladies, do come in and help put some life into the conversation around the bar. Cigars, of course, are optional.

* * *

Chapter 1
Admission Requirements

It's been five years since I've had a prostate, and I miss it the way I miss my youth—as a melancholy reminder of what was, rather than what isn't; a time of endless possibilities, reduced now to limited dreams. Call it wistful thinking.

I can't say I didn't think about my prostate before I decided to get rid of it; I had no choice. Almost every day, there was, and continues to be, enough media attention on prostate cancer to keep it a top of mind subject—especially if you're a man who's hit fifty, and are aware that it's been more prevalent an occurrence than breast cancer.

The prostate is the touted gland of the 90's and everyone's now free to talk about it. *Time* magazine gave it eight pages and a cover blurb. The tabloids feature it as one of the top ten diseases you'd want some South American dictator to acquire. Even a condo neighbor, a man whose name I can't even recall, sidles up to me in the elevator and asks me if I've read about Merv Griffin's having been diagnosed with *it*. "Yeah, his PSA was pretty high," I respond. *Of course, I'd read the stupid article!* Even without a prostate, even as I write this account, I am still drawn to any print or broadcast piece that even hints of a prostate mention. Just because you're discharged from the battle, however scarred but alive, doesn't mean you stop following the news from the front. If anything, you follow it even more assiduously. You know people are out there fighting for every prostate, and well, attention must be paid. You're as drawn to prostate cancer news as a hemorrhoid sufferer is to yet another ad touting relief.

You can now, also, openly fret and stew about the inadequacy of male plumbing design. Couldn't another place for the prostate been found? But alas, as a friend once commented: "God's specialty was humanity, not urology." So there's only so much bitching you can engage in on that subject.

You can, if you wanted to scare the crap out of yourself, contemplate what it would be like if you were diagnosed as having prostate cancer. You can even make believe it won't happen to you. But, like a junky, you can never get enough of that prostate update fix. You're forever hoping—even the survivors—to achieve that eternal high, to read the headline that blisses you out forever, the one that proclaims: Prostate Cancer Cured!

That my father had prostate problems (I think), and that genetic influences can decide whether prostates survive the long haul or not, also lay somewhere in my mind. The reason I'm not sure of whether my father's prostate was on the fritz is because my family, like so many others, never invoked the dreaded C-word (or the P-word, for that matter) except in whispers and in the most roundabout way lest the mere mention of the word somehow mark them, dooming them to an early and unimaginably awful death. But somewhere in his 80's, my father allowed as how he had had something wrong "back there," and that a doctor had done something "up there," but now everything was okay. Where exactly "back there" was, and what was done "up there" and why, I never really learned. But from the way he waved his hand toward his buttocks when he told me about his problem, I suspected that he was talking about his prostate. And while suspicion isn't solid evidence, his hearsay testimony was convincing enough for me; I accepted the fact that genetically, my prostate wouldn't go the 100,000 miles the brochure promised.

I was also made aware of my prostate at each annual physical I endured, courtesy of my then places of employ. From my early fifties on, each visit ended with the digital goose and the litany: "It's getting a little bigger . . . normal for your age . . . nothing to worry about." Different doctors each year; same script for a decade.

Then, in my late fifties, I began to experience symptoms of what I later learned was called Benign Prostatic Hyperplasia (BPH for short)—a common, non-threatening, yet nagging condition: the constant urge to urinate, especially at night; difficulty starting what was usually a diminished stream; a nagging drip after going that forced you to tear off a piece of toilet tissue before you started to urinate so you'd have something to sop up the dripping with—insidious and uncomfortable reminders that your prostate was enlarging, tightening up on the urethra like a clamp on a hose, and would continue to be a constant, annoying presence.

And yet my PSA (prostate specific antigen, for long) scores remained well within the normal range, and no doctor's finger ever detected any unusual outcroppings that might indicate anything was amiss.

When I was almost sixty-one years of age, I became even more intimately acquainted with this obstreperous gland. On March 30, 1994, I was informed that my prostate was cancerous.

My primary care provider was (and still is) Gerald Dominguez, a Tampa, Florida, and board certified internist with a sub-specialty in gastroenterology. (I hate the term "internist;" it leaves me wondering if they neglect to notice your outsides.)

It was the twenty-first of February, 1994, at the second "report" visit of my annual physical and I wasn't listening all that hard. I felt strong and energetic and besides, was accustomed to, and fully expected to hear, "Your heart's strong, lungs are clear, blood pressure is that of a twenty-year old," the usual. But as I was reaching down to pick up my bag, ready to dash, Doctor Dominguez looked up from his reports and said, "Your PSA's doubled. Last year it was three point seven, this year it's seven point five. I don't like that. I want you to see a urologist." It wasn't just his words that affected me. Dominguez's voice, normally a warm, southern comfort alto, had transposed into a chilly baritone, and it was that vocal shift of gears, even more than what was actually said, that I found disturbing.

When I asked what urologist he'd recommend, without a pause, he pointed at the door. "Down the hall," he ordered. "Doctor Mawn. He's good." Dominguez wasn't long on explanations. When he spoke, he expected you to listen. I went down the hall and set up an appointment before leaving the building.

Actually, I'd seen Doctor Mawn the year before. Dominguez had sent me to him after I'd asked whether Proscar or some other prostate-shrinking drug might provide some relief of my irksome urinary symptoms.

At that time, Mawn had me fill out a questionnaire that asked for a ranking of my urinary problems. After he went over the numbers, he allowed as how I wasn't a candidate for such drugs though I was no doubt symptomatic, but on the mild end of the symptom scale, with basically nothing to worry about. He didn't forget to add that if my wee hour wee-wees became more numerous, or if any of the other symptoms became too uncomfortable, I should consult with him again.

It was a cursory sort of visit, yet I didn't feel put off. The question had been answered. I was okay. Nothing to dwell on.

My impression of Doctor Mawn at that time, I confess, is a little spotty. The visit wasn't an urgent one; more of attending to personal things I never seemed to find the time for until my semi-retirement. But I do remember liking him. He was open, professional, and his smile had mensch written all over it.

DAYBOOK ENTRY, 10/5/92
Patient: *Bert Gottlieb; Age: 59*
PSA: *3.7 (per Dr. Dominguez's lab results)*

DRE (digital rectal exam): *Prostate appears Grade II-III enlarged, symmetrical and non-indurated, i.e., did not feel hard or nodular, with no discernible bulkiness or unevenness.*

Reason for Visit: *Inquiring about prostate-shrinking drug treatment (currently given heavy press coverage and advertising) for his BPH symptoms (up 2-3 times a night, some hesitancy when bladder is full). Patient filled out the AUA Symptom Score* to determine if he was a candidate for Proscar, but his tally of only "7" indicated urinary symptoms too mild to qualify for drug treatment.*

Recommendation: *If symptoms become more unpleasant and/or more frequent, to call for an appointment.*

Post Visit Thoughts & Observations: *Initial impression: patient is a New Yorker without a New York attitude, interested in hearing what the doctor knows rather than telling the doctor what he knows—an all too common occurrence, not confined to New Yorkers. He is a critical listener with a seeming abundance of gray matter, but chooses to hold back on the many aspects of life he obviously knows about, staying inside his personal armor until he's sure it's safe to come out.*

At our next meeting on March fifteenth—the one I'd set up when I left Doctor Dominguez's office—Doctor Mawn and I became more intimately acquainted. His digital rectal exam was unlike any I had had before. It was considerably more probing, and though supremely uncomfortable, was so seemingly thorough and focused, I found I was being comforted by the thought that if any finger knew what it was about, Mawn's did.

---

* *Prepared by a select panel of specialists chosen by the American Urologic Association to quantify symptom complaints of men experiencing prostatism (the other medical term for BPH), it consists of seven questions, each one graded from 1 to 5 in terms of severity. The most symptomatic patients would score in the high 30s.*

Of course, I told myself that nothing would be found. My fantasy allowed as how my PSA results were a false alarm—the result of sexual activity or other bodily functionings that can cause PSA numbers to spike upward. That was the dream. The reality proved otherwise when the doctor told me he'd felt a nodule.

I don't know if I showed any signs of reaction to what I'd heard, but my head was screaming. *A nodule? What medical euphemism is "nodule" meant to cover? A protuberance, a knob, a knot like mass of tissue? Dear God! A nodule, a nodule—my kingdom for no nodule! My impulse was to flee.*

Mawn did his best to de-alarm me.

"It could be tumorous tissue, Bert . . . *or* it could be a benign calcified lump of some kind. Nothing to get upset about yet." He paused to look over his glasses at me. "But we do have to go a little further to see what's what."

This was all said so evenly, I convinced myself, at least for a few seconds, that my odds stood at fifty-fifty. Hell, I'd once passed a calcified kidney stone. Perhaps, even as we spoke, excess calcium crystals were forming on the outer edge of my wayward gland. *And maybe there really are extra-terrestrial life forms looking to have their way with us!*

"What does 'further' mean?" I heard my mouth asking, my mind frantically looking for an exit back to a few minutes earlier.

"We have to do a sonogram and a biopsy," Mawn answered. "Annette will set up an appointment for you."

I remember nodding dully, trying to look sage. The sonogram didn't sound so bad (little did I know), but the thought of a biopsy sent another squirt of adrenalin into an already overloaded system. I couldn't wait to leave and be alone so that my innards would quiet down and I could begin to chew on this new turn of events.

DAYBOOK ENTRY, 3/15/94

<u>*Patient:*</u> *Bert Gottlieb*   *Age: 60+*

<u>*PSA:*</u> *7.5* *(Doubled in the 1 1/2 years since first visit, now out of normal range.)*

<u>*DRE:*</u> *Revealed a nodule on the right posterior lateral lobe of the capsule with an estimated size of 1 1/2 centimeters (about 3/4").*

<u>*Reason for Visit:*</u> *Significant change in PSA level (detected initially by Dr. Dominguez's lab work during annual examination).*

<u>*Recommendation:*</u> *Further examination via transrectal ultrasound imaging with ultrasonic-guided biopsy.[1] (Prescribed Maxaquin 400 mg. prior to procedure.)*

<u>*Post Visit Thoughts & Observations:*</u> *Patient has met the two criteria (elevated PSA, positive DRE) to justify proceeding with continued testing. He obviously understands that these next test steps are necessary, and that until the results are in, no conclusions can be drawn. In spite of his outer calm, his concern is evident.*

I came home with no recall of how I got there.

"How did it go?" Rose, my infinitely better half, asked.

I didn't answer her straight off. Instead, I put my keys and bag down, and then feigned having to go to the bathroom so I could figure out how to put the best light on this nodule business.

"So what's up?" she asked as I came back into the room.

"The doctor felt a lump. Could be nothing. A calcified something-or-other. He has to run a couple of tests to check it out." I offered this neutral version of events as if I were reading a news summary off a teleprompter..

"And if it's not a calcium something-or-other?" Rose would have made a great prosecuting attorney.

"He's not sure," I lied. "That's why the tests."

"What kind of tests?" I tried to sound casual. "Oh, a

sonogram and a . . . a tissue sample."

"You mean a biopsy."

"Yeah, a biopsy." I started to sag.

"So it might be cancer."

"It might be. You never know," I lied.

"True, you never know." Rose now lied.

After over 30 years of marriage, couples know when to close it off, when to quit the field; know there'll be another time to kick the subject around. We squeezed our hands together and smiled bravely, if wryly, at each other.

"How're you doing?" Rose asked softly.

I shrugged. "Okay, I guess." Lying again.

We squeezed hands even tighter. There wasn't much more to say just then. Since my prostate was in limbo until the sonogram-biopsy, life decided to add a dash more spice to my medical stew in the form of a rash so exquisitely itchy, I couldn't stop scratching until I had torn the skin and drawn blood. The day after I saw Doctor Mawn, I went to see a dermatologist.

The rash had started sometime after Doctor Dominguez had told me about my elevated PSA.

The skin doctor, who shall remain nameless to avoid any litigation, was a beaming, jovial man. He took scrapings from the back of my thighs, where the rash was most apparent, and started to leave (I assumed) to peer at my cells under a microscope to determine what exactly the rash was. But as he started out the door, he reminded himself to ask me if there were any other places the rash had manifested itself.

"On my elbows and forearms. Mostly on the elbows," I said.

Hearing that, had he not been holding his scrapings, I was sure he would have jumped up and clicked his heels, so elated was he at this seemingly wonderful bit of information. "Ooh," he clucked. "You've really helped with the diagnosis." And out he went to, I

17

imagined, a small office lab, for a close-up inspection of my cellular detritus.

When he came back, he was as exultant as if he had discovered a cure for terminal acne. "I was right," he crowed. "When you told me it was on your elbows, I thought it was psoriasis. And it is." He was elated. In spite of having just delivered a curse on his patient's head, elbows, and who knew where else, he was depressingly elated.

My adrenal glands were given a good workout that week, pumping a goodly measure of distress into my system for the second day in a row.

Psoriasis. I could see myself covered with thickening, white, scaly lesions. Even if this prostate business turned out to be a false alarm (which I somehow doubted), I now had one of the worst imaginable skin conditions short of leprosy. My heart broke.

"This should help the itching," Doctor Elated said brightly, handing me a prescription for some sort of ointment. I could have killed him. But how do you kill your uncle? How do you do away with someone so inordinately cheerful he could convince an atheist there really was a Santa Claus?

"What did Doctor Dermatology have to say?" Rose asked too casually.

"That it's psoriasis," I answered too glumly, because she jumped up from where she was sitting and hustled me over to a window.

"Let's see," she commanded, kneeling behind me and slapping my outer thigh, the universal married couples signal that means, "*Drop your pants.*"

After staring at my skin close up, she slapped my thigh again (the "up pants" signal), and opined from her crouch, "Doesn't look like psoriasis to me."

"Since when did you become an expert on skin diseases?" I screamed. She ignored the uncharacteristic outburst, looked at me as if I were mentally challenged, and quietly said, "It's not psoriasis."

I went over to the bookshelves and dug out our copy of *The Merck Manual*, a desk drawer ready-reference for many doctors. Granted, it was the '72 edition, and that in '94, it would have seen immense changes in medical diagnosis and therapy in dozens of areas, but inasmuch as there were still a plethora of small-space ads dotting the newspapers, touting cures for this grim condition, I doubted that psoriasis had seen much upgrading since the earlier printing, maybe not since the flood.

I read the requisite section, but when I came to the words " . . . complete and permanent remission is rare . . . no therapeutic method assures a cure," I could have cried.

Why me? What sins am I suffering for? Is this the Curse of Three? Three on a match? Three strikes and you're out? First it's the old prostate! Now it's psoriasis! What "p" was next? Pneumonia? Parkinson's? Planned Parenthood?

It was a short paranoia-induced riff playing itself out, courtesy of garden variety fear, more commonly called peeing in one's pants.

To temper what I had just read, Rose, who had come over and was reading along with me, pointed to a sentence in the diagnosis section that ended with, ". . . may be confused with over half a dozen other skin conditions. In doubtful cases, biopsy usually establishes the diagnosis."

I wondered if a scraping was the same as a biopsy.

"What?" Rose asked, reading my mind.

"I was wondering if a scraping qualifies as a biopsy."

"A biopsy is a tissue sample. The doctor scraped off tissue. Ipso facto, a scraping is a biopsy. Or would you have felt better if he dug out a hunk of flesh?"

"If the biopsy said psoriasis, that's what its gotta be....- Unless . . . " I tried to shake the thought.

"Unless what?" Rose asked, Marcia Clark badgering a witness.

"Unless, when I told the good doctor, or nutty professor if you prefer, that it was on my elbows, he was so convinced I had psoriasis, he never bothered or forgot to check the tissue samples, maybe got busy with other patients, and by the time he came back, I had psoriasis, no doubt about it, yessirree!"

While I was embracing this lunatic thought, Rose took out our copy of the American Medical Association's *Family Medical Guide*, turned to a page of photographic color plates and, pointing to the largest illustration, said, "You don't look anything like that."

To which I trumped her ace by declaring, a bit too fervently, "That's because mine just started. Give it time and I'll be the poster boy for the goddamned disease."

Rose backed off. I was obviously in a state of acceptance.

I went to sleep that night counting "pees." Somewhere between presbyopia and priapism I finally nodded off.

Itching, night sweats and the all-too familiar frequency of urination at night* made for a rocky rest that night and the countless others that were to follow.

On Monday, March 28th, my day starts earlier than it's supposed to. Even though the sonogram-biopsy appointment isn't until 10:00 AM, anticipation rouses me at 5:00 AM.

I pad out to the kitchen to prepare a cup of tea, pop my prescribed

---

*The medical term for this condition is nocturia. The thing is, when you utter the word, it's as if you're summoning some mythical goddess, a magical princess of the evening. What you get is a haridan who wrenches you up from bed, points a too-long fingernail at the bathroom and shrieks, "Take a piss!" And when the stream is slow to start, "What's taking you so long?" *Nocturia:* too beautiful a word to describe so ugly a condition. Let's vote to change the name and give Nocturia back to her rightful place antibiotics, figure out that I have to take a Fleet enema at around 8:00 AM, and am reminded from the detailed prep sheet Doctor Mawn's office provided, that I have to drink a quart of fluid—within fifteen minutes time—an hour prior to my appointment. It is necessary, the instructions say, to have a full bladder for the ultrasound examination. I'll bet.

It's still dark outside, the night terrors haven't gone to bed yet, and I'm alone, feeling an urgency in my bladder that shouldn't be there yet. A mess is what I am, and it's only 5:10 AM.

When it's time for the Fleet enema, what should be a mildly unpleasant experience, instead, dredges up early emotions that churn my insides before the process has even begun.

Kneeling on a bath mat, head on the floor, ready to insert the vaselined tip, I'm a child again, forced to submit, a naked sinner praying (begging, really) that this time I be spared the indignity, and more important, the awful stomach cramping that enemas bring on. So unhinged am I, that as the pain spreads through my bowels, I even calculate whether I'm at least facing East.

A second cup of tea, the remainder of my morning ablutions, and daylight, each help to lift my spirits and carry me to 9:00 AM. All that remains is to down the required quart.

As I pour the first glassful, my bladder tingles in anticipation, while I stand there wishing I had learned to chugalug.

"Mister Gottlieb?"

I nod at the cheerful, young technical specialist as I come into one of Doctor Mawn's examining rooms. "I'm going to do your ultrasound test today," she informs me.

"No doctor?" I ask, voice shaky.

She hands me an open-backed examining gown. "Oh, he'll be in in a little while. We have to get you ready first. You can leave your socks on," she adds as she leaves the room.

I disrobe quickly, even though at my age, embarrassment is harder to come by, and over the years I've grown enough personal armor to be able to duck inside when the going gets to the blush stage. I understand, too, that the technician is trained to handle the undressing moment delicately. I picture her standing behind the door, intent on the sweep second hand of her watch, waiting patiently until it reaches the proper elapsed time so she can return without catching me with my pants down around my ankles.

Tying up the gown is the hardest part of the disrobing exercise because it has to be done backwards, and as everybody knows, the "behind-your-back-skills" gene is not carried on the male chromosome the way color-blindness is. Simply put, a man cannot do this task.

Having checked to see if I am decent, and noting that I am merely in one of the backward-knotting, shoulder-dislocating positions, Miss Technical Specialist comes back into the room, checks her equipment, fondles what resembles a large, gray marital aid, then beckons me to lie on my side on the examining table.

As she fusses with the pillows under my head, I want to remind her that my head isn't the part of me that will need comfort if that jumbo-sized vibrator is going to be introduced inside me.

Thankfully, I'm facing away from the action, as if I'm on one side of the room, my behind on the other. But from that position I can't watch the monitor with its jerky black and white picture of my prostate, and so can't make futile attempts at humor, which always buoys my spirits and masks my agitation. *Is it a boy or a girl, doctor?*

"I want you to relax now," she tells my behind. "the more you can relax, the less uncomfortable it will be." Sure. As soon as elephants learn to fly.

It is, indeed, uncomfortable, but not painful. It is also awkward and unnatural, an act of intrusion profoundly unsettling. (Unless, of course, you're so inclined.)

I do my Zen best to relax, but find myself gritting my teeth. "How're you doin'?" Doctor Mawn asks coming into the room, the answer apparent in his understanding grimace.

"I thought you were going to miss the party!" I respond a bit too cheerily, a lame-humored thank-you to him for acknowledging my distress.

He squeezes my shoulder, consults with the technician, then both of them go out of the room, and I'm left with the probe hanging out of me. It's pressing on the area that seems to control rectal "winking", and no matter how I wiggle or try to relax, my rectum is in constant spasm trying to expel it. If the doctor and his technician don't come in soon, I envision the probe shooting out of me and dropping onto the floor, rendering it useless, and the morning but a rehearsal for another big opening.

Moments away from my wresting the probe out of its hiding place, the doctor and technician come back in. They are all concentration, guiding the probe, whispering words to each other as if announcing a golf game on TV.

"This may sting a bit," Doctor Mawn warns my backside. The probe is twisted and turned until both seem happy with what they see on the video monitor, and then there's a tiny, sharp bite deep inside me. Some fussing over slides. More probe wriggling and whispering. Then another bite. Then more. And now the doctor is helping me into a sitting position, studying my face. I let out a breath I hadn't realized I'd been holding. I don't try to stand up, my knees know better. He squeezes my shoulder reassuringly. I try to smile.

DAYBOOK ENTRY, 3/28/94
Patient: Bert Gottlieb
Reason for Visit: Transrectal ultrasound/biopsy
DRE prior to the biopsy revealed a hypoechogenic area approxi-

mately 1 cm., noted on the transverse side that corresponded to the palpable nodule. Extracted 6 tissue samples in and around the suspect area. Initial examination revealed an image of less dense appearance (or "hypoechoic", as radiologists call this echo reflection). Pathology lab results to quantify.

(Estimated prostate volume: 70 grams; PSA Density: 0.106)

<u>Post Visit Thoughts & Observations:</u> After the procedure, Bert's color and good humor returned rather quickly, considering the process is, in the words of even the renowned Dr. Patrick Walsh, "not much fun." It is an unnatural and unpleasant experience, but it's rarely painful, and usually well-tolerated.

Though not major surgery, a biopsy is invasive, and as such, complications may arise, which is why a cleansing enema is called for beforehand, with antibiotics taken both before and after the procedure to fight off possible infections. Of course, minor rectal bleeding can occur, and/or a trace of blood may be found in semen, but both complications are rare and usually temporary, clearing up by themselves.

The development of the spring-loaded biopsy gun has made this procedure simpler and safer—and guided by the ultrasound image—far surer. When the physician has everything lined up, he can aim the tip of the biopsy needle and squeeze the trigger, confident he's on target. Once fired, a small needle shoots through the rectal wall (where there are few nerve endings to register pain) and springs back with a small core of tissue approximately one millimeter thick—enough for the pathologist to examine for abnormalities.

Doubtless, there will be, in the near future, a quantum leap in testing procedures, resulting in ever-fewer biopsies, but for now and possibly forever, we must examine actual tissue samples for conclusive proof of prostate cancer.

This time, the drive home is real enough; no moments lost to mental flights of panic with its accompanying trip amnesia. This time, I can admire the silver-tipped waters of Tampa Bay, the stately rows of palm trees, the sky masked by clouds, the sun streaming through the few spaces left for it to squeeze through, a painting by Tiepolo come to life. I can appreciate all this scenery with incredible clarity because what I can't do is sit, unless perching on one hip, body tilted to one side, can be called sitting. Navigating an interstate in this off-center position (with an occasional cheek shift thrown in for good measure), and at well above the lawful limit, sharpens the senses and gets you to see things you rarely notice anymore. I sensed my eyes would stay wide open from here on. If life is "a dome of many-colored glass," as Shelley wrote, I was going to make sure I never lost sight of its magnificence once this bad dream was over.

After a hot bath and a cold martini, I was confident my spirits as well as my rectum would be in better shape, and I'd be free to wonder what life would be like after my next visit to Doctor Mawn, two days hence.

Daybook Entry, 3/29/94

Patient: *Bert Gottlieb*
Lab Results: Positive indication of moderately-differentiated adenocarcinoma, Gleason-scored at 6 (3+3).
Post Visit Thoughts & Observations: *The Gleason Grading System, originally devised in 1977 by Doctor Lawrence Gleason, a pathologist and prostate cancer researcher, indicates how aggressively the tumor appears to be developing based on its cellular architecture.[2]*

Tissue samples are Gleason-graded on a scale of one to five—one being the least and five the worst, or most aggressive-looking.[3]

A low Gleason score indicates that cell architecture is well-differentiated and that prognosis is quite good no matter what, if anything, is done; a high score indicates poor differentiation with a gloomy outlook no matter what, or how combative the therapy. Luckily, Bert's cancer fell between the two extremes.

The next step after determining the grade of his tumor was to ascertain the clinical "stage" of his cancer, since, more than any other factor, staging[4] guides us to the most appropriate treatment options and probable outcome.

However, having decided on a clinical stage is not an assumption carved in stone. It is merely a working hypothesis based on information from the diagnostic tests. It's a little like having to diagnose a car's ailments without being able to peak under the hood. Yet in spite of the inability to fully look at the patient's engine, physicians do a fairly good job of staging, though in a significant percentage of cases, however, clinical understaging occurs, the physician discovering after a prostatectomy that the tumor was a stage higher than originally rated.

In Bert's case, since he is in good physical shape, of the possible treatment options, I couldn't recommend "watchful waiting." Keeping an eye on prostate cancer development is more suitable to the management of older men with low-grade tumors, or men who prefer, for a variety of reasons, not to pursue any further treatment. And Bert did not fit that profile.

Also, the fact that his tumor appeared to be clinically organ-confined meant that hormone manipulation—employing either LHRH (Luteinizing Hormone Releasing Hormone) agonists such as Lupron® (Leoprolide) or Zolade®—would not be a wise choice, since these agents merely slow the rate of tumor growth, but aren't expected to cure.

And in spite of a number of articles in prestigious professional journals showing excellent survival figures for "watchful waiting," and although the figures were legitimately derived, further analysis of the data revealed that the men studied were older, and that the case histories excluded men with higher than average Gleason scores. Since we know the higher the score, the more aggressive the cancer will act, the figures become problematic at best.

This leaves surgery or radiation as the treatment options which offer Bert the best hope for survival. And of the two, at the time of this writing, no one can say with certainty which of them offer the best outcomes.[5]

Having said that, it should be noted that there is an informal, though general consensus amongst urologists, oncologists and even radiotherapists, that the younger the patient, the more they tend to recommend a radical prostatectomy, which is the total removal of the prostate and seminal vesicles. After discussing radiation procedures as a viable option, I am still going to recommend the "radical" to Bert as the first choice. His choice will, naturally, depend on how he feels about radiation treatments (after a consultation with a radiotherapist, which I will also recommend), and/or his willingness to accept the risks and the possible serious consequences of this major operation.

CHAPTER FOOTNOTES

1.   The development of high quality ultrasound equipment is the second most important technologic advance (the first is PSA testing) in accurately locating the suspicious portion of the gland, helping to precisely guide the biopsy needle to the target, where previously, the urologist's fingertip was the only available tool for discerning the suspicious area. Yet even with the most experienced finger and a thorough knowledge of anatomy, it was, at best, a hit or miss process, not unlike trying to thread a needle blindfolded. Today, the sonar-type image derived from the ultrasound machine is similar to how the fetus is viewed in the mother's womb, with the outlines and dimensions of the prostate easily recognizable, and with tumors appearing as lighter or darker spots. (Normal prostate tissue is seen as a medium gray on the sonogram monitor.)

The ultrasound picture is also a better means of estimating the "volume" of the prostate which, when divided into the PSA score, provides a better idea of PSA density—another indication of the likelihood of adenocarcinoma (the formal medical term for prostate cancer). The rule of thumb is: the PSA density number should not be more than 15% of the volume of the prostate. But rules are made to be broken, since density is but one of many factors that are taken into consideration by the urologist.

PSA "velocity" is, like the PSA density factor, yet a further variation of PSA testing procedures. In this case, the rate of PSA change is charted on a continuum rather than waiting for a man's PSA to arrive at a reading of 4, since adenocarcinoma causes PSA to rise faster than BPH. So if there is an average consistent increase from three readings taken over a period of a year and a half, PSA levels having tripled (from, say, as low as 1.1 to a not too high 3.7), further investigation would clearly be called for, since a PSA rise which registers above the curve normally seen as men age, is worrisome, and perhaps evidence of a worsening condition.

The reason the PSA test is the premier breakthrough of the last decade is because it is a proven tumor marker. In most cases, the larger the tumor, the higher the PSA, and thus the greater need for continued testing.

In spite of some of the controversy surrounding PSA testing and its early warning system, we are discovering prostate cancer soon enough to provide treatment, since delay can compromise the effectiveness of any treatment, and since, in curable stages, prostate cancer seldom produces symptoms. Thanks to PSA technology, we have jumped a hundred years forward in the last ten. And with advances in the field being made almost daily, it isn't difficult to imagine another hundred year leap in, hopefully, only five years, with PSA tests becoming even more acute and definitive, making early detection even more predictable, and today's tests archaic by comparison.

An important refinement to PSA evaluation is the free PSA/ Total PSA ratio.It has been known for some time that there tends to be a relatively higher ratio of free PSA in men with BPH, as compared to men with prostate cancer. A prospective, definitive, multi-institutional study* composed of 733 men who had negative DREs and or PSAs between 4 and 10 Ng/ml, clearly demonstrated that using a cut-off of 25% Free PSA/ Total PSA, that 95% of prostate cancers would be detected, sparing 20% of the men whose biopsies would have been negative. Applied to a large population, this would result in tremendous savings and discomfort, without adversely affecting the percentages of cancer detection.

*Catalona, W.J.; Partinaw, et al—Use of the Percentage of Free PSA to Enhance Differentiation of Prostate Cancer from BPH. A prospective multicenter clinical trial.*JAMA*, 1998; 279 (19) 1542-1547.

2.   Healthy prostate cells are round or oblong, with smooth edges.

They are evenly-spaced, their nuclei small, and are well-differentiated. Cancer cells have irregular or jagged edges, with nuclei that take up the entire cell, and are not well-differentiated. And the less well-differentiated the cells look, the more aggressive the cancer usually is.

3   The pathologist assigns Gleason grades to the two most abundant types, which numbers are then added together. Example: a Gleason score of 2+3 would mean that the most abundant cells were graded as a 2, and the next most common as a 3, for a score of 5.

4   It is achieved using either of two equivalent systems: the Jewett-Whitmore (ABCD) Scale, or the International TNM (Tumor, Node and Metastasis) Scale. Since Bert's prostate contained a 1½ centimeter palpable nodule, I determined his clinical stage to be B on the Jewett-Whitmore Scale and clinical stage TB_2NoMo on the TNM Scale (TB describes the cancer, with the number indicating its size; No is shorthand for "no regional lymph node metastasis"; and Mo stands for "no distant metastasis.")

Thus, either type of staging is the synthesis of tumor size, location and whether it's confined or extending through the prostate capsule.

The reason I stress clinical staging, is because there is another type of staging: pathological. Clinical staging is based on physical findings and X-ray or other imaging studies such as CT scan or ultrasound. Pathological staging is based on the findings found at surgery—what the surgeon and pathologist actually see in and on the organs upon examination.

5   A few years ago, a blue ribbon panel of academic urologists and statisticians was put together to review all the available treatment literature and come up with a definitive conclusion as to which treat-

ment was best. The panel wisely agreed on inclusion and exclusion criteria before they analyzed anything. They excluded: nonproductive studies, studies with inconsequential populations, studies with questionable statistical methodology, and all anecdotal studies. Included, though, were nearly 10,000 papers from all over the world. These were winnowed down to 1,000, which were in turn, reviewed and further narrowed down to around 100 reliable study references.

After much discussion, the conclusion was that there really wasn't enough hard data to conclusively recommend surgery over radiation, or vice versa.

Even before the panel reached its conclusion, it was apparent that longitudinal-prospective studies were needed, and indeed these are ongoing, with results expected in a few years. Which doesn't help someone who has been diagnosed with prostate cancer last week.

Chapter 2
Enrollment Rules

It is, at last, the afternoon of March thirtieth, the day we are to hear the results of the biopsy. Rose has been invited to this meeting, which not only doesn't bode well for what's in store, it chagrins me to think that anyone could imagine me needing support. Short of hearing I have months to live, I didn't need anyone to lean on in case the news was so bad my knees began to head for the floor. I can faint on my own, thank you.

I may be sixty-one, but there's a much younger person living inside me. He's got the reckless confidence of his salad days. He truly believes he is indestructible, this foolish, callow lad does.

Besides, it's my prostate, mine alone—the part of me that will ultimately be sliced, diced and otherwise dealt with. If it's gone south, whether someone's at my side or not, it and me share the same cabin on this trip, and it's only got one bed. Contrarily, I'm glad Rose is with me, but the uncertainty of what lies ahead crowds out any conversation she and I may have had on the drive into Tampa. Our minds are too busy picking apart daisies, hoping he has it not.

Time has become a contradictory element: on the one hand, it seems to be moving at warp speed, blurring every picture I've taken on this inexorable journey; conversely, it feels as if it's crawling, dragging all the demons into slow-motion focus so I'm face to face with their every hideous feature. My clock is obviously in need of a screw tightening.

When Rose and I walk into Doctor Mawn's waiting room, it could be the lobby of a retirement home for aged prostates. Dour older men (and what I assume to be their life companions) fill the chairs, waiting their turn with the doctor. No chatter breaks the stillness, no eyes connect with any other; everyone is inside themselves, safe for the moment in their private agonies.

I find myself reading the same sentence in a dated *Newsweek*. Every so often a couple comes out a side door in the waiting room, more grim and quiet than when they went in. I hurt for them. I hurt for me—us. I wish it were tomorrow and the waiting was over. If only this was a dream.

After the obligatory urine sample and another long wait, we are eventually ushered into the doctor's office—all black leather and dark wood, a large banker's desk occupying most of the space—a place to deposit your hopes, or perhaps borrow some at a decent interest rate.

"Sorry it took so long," Doctor Mawn apologizes as he joins us. I wave it off because it is not a pro forma expression of regrets; he means it. His body language informs me that, in his time, he's done his share of waiting and understands the numbing of the spirit that waiting inflicts. It is also evident; that while he tries his damnedest to stay on schedule, there's no way he can calculate his time precisely. I understand this and am reassured by it. This is not a man who slyly checks his watch to ensure he's running on time. Mawn will be late on occasion because, I sense, short cuts and short shrift are not his style, that his best shot is his only one, even if it runs the clock out. I know this as I know my name. I know too, that there are times you've got to take the measure of a man and trust your calculations, and that this is one of those times.

"I gather," he says, checking his notes, "This is Rose." The warmth of his shy smile thaws Rose and she smiles back, the tightness in her lips gone. I see this as a good start, because if Rose doesn't cotton to someone in that first millisecond of meeting, I know to chalk him or her off the list. Rose's instincts are unerring, and I heed them even more than I do my own.

With the other shoe about to drop, and in spite of the fact that I am sure of what we will hear and have never been a gambler, I'm betting that my odds are good. Also lighting candles, just in case.

Doctor Mawn gets right to it. "Bert, the biopsy reveals a malignancy." I've crapped out.

For the next few minutes *malignancy* is all I hear. It resounds in my head, echoing so violently I can barely make out what the doctor's answers are to questions I seem to be throwing at him—a torrent of words to block out that one word, that unthinkable, poisonous, scarifying word.

At the same time, a terribly loud drumming begins, and in shrill neon, the words *prostate cancer* dance across my eyes. The headache is just beginning.

At my insistence, and in spite of his reluctance, since he prefers to wait a week or so to outline the options, Doctor Mawn carefully lays out each of the treatment possibilities.

What I remember is this: first line of defense, with a 95% recovery rate, is surgical removal of the prostate—the radical prostatectomy, or "radical" as the medical fraternity shorthands it. Which will result in loss of seminal vesicles, the glands that provide the fluid component to a man's ejaculate. The result of that loss was best described by George Burns when, in his early 90's, he was queried about his sexual output. "I come dust," he blithely answered. Point being, the lack of seminal vesicles doesn't impair the ability to experience orgasm; there's just no ejaculate—the ultimate example of a dry hump. Upside: kiss wet spots on the sheets goodbye. That is, if the other possible downsides—impotence (fifty-fifty odds) and incontinence (10% chance)—don't befall you.

Two forms of radiation therapy are then put on the table: one which involves getting bombarded five times a week for eight or so weeks, with especially uncomfortable side effects, but with a 95%

remission rate; the other approach consists of the implantation of radioactive seeds directly into the prostate, where they, in effect, burn out the malignant tissue. Pluses: a 95% cure rate and but a day's stay in the hospital. Minuses: up to a 50% probability of impotency, a 5% chance of persistent rectal bleeding, and possible incontinence. And if either radiation procedure is a failure, forget going back. Any attempt to perform a "radical" at this point is considered a salvage operation due to the high incidence of morbidity that results. "I wouldn't do it," Mawn says, allowing as how while other doctors might, his tone infers that it is a moral and ethical consideration, and that he stands on the side of the angels.

Alternative medicine, including hormone treatments, holistic approaches and unproven therapies are presented as a package which we're invited to explore if we are of a mind to, but which Mawn confesses he doesn't put much clinical stock in. I'm inclined to agree, because even though I've been a lifelong Democrat, I suddenly realize that liberalism is incompatible with prostate cancer. I'm voting for a Newt or a Pat in this election.

Last on the list is "watchful waiting," a Scandinavian import which consists of merely checking the prostate, with the thought that you'll die from something else before your prostate rolls over you. What a smorgasbord of unappetizing choices.

"Tom, if you were me," I ask, using his proper name for the first time, feeling, I suspect, that at this point, we should be communicating on a less hierarchical, more intimate basis. "What would *you* do, considering everything you know about my condition?"

I had already ruled out watching and waiting to see what I would die from. Considering the possible side effects, seeding my rotting prostate with radioactive particles was also ruled out. So were the many clinically unverifiable alternative approaches. I knew, too, that Tom's answer would be biased; he was a surgeon and operate is what surgeons do. But I also knew that any bias would be leavened by ethical and professional considerations. I was also questioning whether this wasn't akin to asking a fox to guard your chickens.

"If I were you, I would get it out," Tom answers without hesitation. "But," he quickly adds, "there's no need to make up your mind about any one treatment right away. Your kind of prostate cancer is very slow growing. Probably been developing for maybe three or four years. You can take your time to make up your mind with no harm. But I do want you to consult with a radiologist, see what he has to say. And please feel free to get a second opinion—in fact, I really recommend it—before you make up your mind."

With the guessing over, and the prayers rendered worthless, reality has a chance to enter the fray, and surprisingly, provides a calming effect. It is, it comes to me, the not knowing that distorts things; facts can be dealt with. Guesses, like ghosts, are insubstantial, yet frightening in their ability to metamorphose into whatever form your fears imagine. Knowledge opens the windows and lets in the light.

I suddenly feel a hunger to swallow up as much information about prostate cancer as I can stomach.

I reach over and squeeze Rose's hand, a gesture meant to communicate that everything is going to be all right, that I am okay with this turn of events, steady as she goes, stiff upper lip, all of that. But the message doesn't reach her. Rose is in some other hell, contemplating her own demons. As bad as I feel for myself, I feel even worse for her. From now on, I know I'll have to be braver than I've ever been to lighten the load I'm sure she will be carrying until this business is concluded.

Since my appetite for facts hasn't begun to be sated, I ask Tom what the medical community thinks is the cause of this seeming upsurge in prostate cancer; whether PSA tests with their early detection capabilities are the cause of the bump in the numbers. I need to start somewhere, but for the moment, that is the only question that comes to mind in spite of the fact that what causes prostate cancer is of far less interest to me than what cures it. None of what I know to be important questions are standing still long enough for me to grab onto one.

"PSA testing's been taken into consideration when they're setting out the statistics," Tom says. "The numbers are just growing. Our best guess is that there are some other environmental influences . . . the water we drink, the food we eat, too much fat in our diets, bovine growth hormones in meat and milk . . . the air we breath . . . something we're ingesting. Frankly, we're not sure." He shakes his head in frustration. "Today, this afternoon, I had to give three patients the same bad news." He winces at the thought. That he feels for all his patients is patently apparent.

Before we exit the office, an appointment is made for me to have a CAT and a bone scan six days hence. These are necessary tests, Tom explains, no matter which treatment option is chosen. They determine if the cancer has migrated to any of the surrounding tissue, or is, hopefully, contained within the confines of the prostate. Another nail biter. These next test results could change the direction I seemed to be headed toward, to yet another, bleak place, one that I couldn't, at that crushing moment, even begin to contemplate.

DAYBOOK ENTRY: 3/30/94

Patient: Bert Gottlieb
Reason for Visit: To hear report of malignancy
Recommendation: Radical prostatectomy if subsequent imaging tests are negative.
Followup: Bone and pelvic CT scan to fully stage the lesion.
Post Visit Thoughts & Observations: Bert took the news in thoughtfully, but it was evident that he was wrestling to control his emotions, holding his feelings at bay until he had heard the

whole story.

His wife, Rose, was concerned and vigilant, recording every word for later playback, when the emotional temperature had cooled and reason was allowed back in.

Neither mate broke down, nor did I expect them to. The Gottliebs are a strong couple, loving life-partners who will make the prudent decisions necessary to survive this shattering experience, whatever comes to pass.

One of the most difficult things a physician must do is tell another human being that they have a life-threatening malignancy. Worse, yet, there is no easy way it can be done. Nevertheless, it is crucial that the task be handled as mindfully and compassionately as possible, knowing the impact of this moment can be as long-lasting as a surgical scar.

Nobody is spared from this visceral wrenching, not even doctors. I have three friends (urologists all) who had been diagnosed positively for prostate cancer. Each underwent a radical prostatectomy. And each of them (and their spouses)—though professionally conversant with prostate cancer and all its physical and emotional complications—were as devastated by this experience as someone learning about it for the first time. Point is, everyone gets shaken, nobody is prepared, and everybody is scared.

Many years ago, at Temple University School of Medicine, a respected professor of internal medicine gave a lecture to my about-to-graduate senior class. The subject: how— and how not to—deliver bad news. His sage advice is as valuable now as it was then, and no doubt, will remain so until bad news ceases to exist.

His first never-to-be-forgotten lesson was that the onerous task of informing the patient must be done solely by the physician. It may not, can not, and should never be delegated to nurses, nursing office assistants, or anyone else. And it must, if possible, be done face to face. Obviously, if the situation is urgent, and someone is out of town and can only be reached by phone, that is next best—but again, only by the doctor.

The professor's next instruction taught us that the physician must be fully aware of every word and gesture he or she makes at that awful moment, because there cannot be any misinterpretation at this point. Denial has a strong pull, and can only be an influence if the message is not well communicated. There is a moral imperative here for the physician to not only know what to say, but how to say it. And it is paramount that the word "cancer," "malignancy," or "carcinoma" (whichever seems appropriate), be used at least once during a bad news session so that the patient can in no way misconstrue the facts.

The classic (and perhaps apocryphal) story told in medical circles, is of a doctor telling a patient that his biopsy was positive. The patient, thinking "positive" meant good news, promptly proceeded to forget about it. It wasn't until a year later that he discovered a positive biopsy meant the presence of cancer. Luckily, his discovery was in time. It could have been too late just as easily.

Once the doctor is confident that the bad news has been digested, it is important to look at the other side of the page, stressing the fact that prostate cancer is not always, and indeed, is usually not, fatal.

After that fact has been absorbed, and hopefully lifted spirits somewhat, the discussion should only then be directed to the "where-do-we-go-from-here?" stage, reminding the patient that further tests and study will be needed anyway, so no decisions have to be made at this time.

Also, at this time, all the available relevant medical literature the physician has on hand should be given to the patient, along with other suggested reading materials. The better informed about his condition, the better able the prostate cancer patient will be to make the upcoming critical choices necessary for his recovery. Knowledge is, indeed, power, and especially where life and its quality is concerned, ignorance should never be an excuse.

Contrarily, a bad news session is not the time for an in-depth discussion of the disease. Lengthy statistical analyses and projected outcomes of the various treatment options are better dealt with at a subsequent meeting. And certainly, no treatment decisions should be made, since the necessary staging studies have not been completed.

There are good reasons for not saying too much. To begin with, it is important for the patient to have time to read the literature, digest the information, and learn as much as possible about his condition. He also needs time to discuss this atomizing turn of events in his life with mate, family and friends. This is not the time in a man's life to clam up, as too many men are prone to do. Rather, it is a time to reach out, facing this adversity with as much knowledge and encouragement a man can get.

Another reason for deferring any decision, is that the patient's primary care physician may not yet be aware of the diagnosis, and his or her input can often be invaluable in determining treatment procedures. If a patient has, for example, extensive cardiovascular or pulmonary disease, certain surgical approaches pose a higher-than-average risk, a fact which must be taken into consideration before any choices are encouraged.

At the conclusion of this visit, a definite return appointment should be set up. Mates and/or other close family members should be encouraged to attend, because at that session, a discussion of all the options and their ramifications will take place,

*hopefully providing enough information to bring the patient closer
to a decision that best suits him and his condition.*

*Bert was an exception to the rule that a bad news session
is not the right time for a drawn-out discussion. I could see that,
in spite of his inner turmoil, he had to know what he was facing
before he left the office. He needed as much data as he could to
chew on, even though he no doubt knew it would taste exceedingly bitter. And so I obliged with enough information to satisfy
his curiosity without overwhelming it. I laid out the options, and
their statistics for intact recovery versus those of incontinence or
impotence. The only thing I glossed over was approaches like
cryosurgery that were, at that time, unproven clinically, and not
fully FDA approved. It was a new and fascinating approach to
the problem, but with insufficient studies under its belt (remember, this was 1994) to even consider offering it as an option. The
concept: freeze the prostate by inserting probes of liquid nitro-
gen into it, and when it thaws, cancer cells will rupture and die,
leaving the rest of the gland intact. But aside from its too short
track record, and its high risk of erectile dysfunction and other
uncomfortable side effects, it was usually reserved for patients
who were unsuitable candidates for surgery or radiation, and that
wasn't Bert.*

*When pressed to answer what I would do if I were in his
shoes, I told him that, barring any problems cropping up in his
next series of tests, I would choose the radical prostatectomy.
And I meant it. But I could see Bert inwardly questioning whether
I was selling and whether he should be buying.*

Rose and I hold hands as we leave Tom's office and ride down the
elevator, bumping into people, doors, oblivious to everyone and everything until we reach the car and are forced to disconnect. But once

the car is started, we again reach out and intertwine our fingers; touching is communication enough at this time. It says everything that needs to be said, and perhaps, many things that shouldn't be given voice to, not at this time, not when our spirits are so bruised. It also holds back the tears that would surely flow if either of us tried to speak. Hands clasped, our silence is a prayer.

The service is over when I break the quiet with, "Let's get drunk!" Rose squeezes my hand; a silent yes and thank you at the same time.

A fistful of tortilla chips swathed in salsa cruda, washed down with several Margaritas and perhaps a couple of amber Dos Equis at Rio Bravo—our Tex-Mex cantina of choice—might not boost our sagging mood, but would certainly go a long way toward dulling the pain.

I even looked forward to a nerve-jangling morning-after in the dim hope that my hungover headache might override the terrible pain my inner self was experiencing. Which is what gave rise to (or perhaps it was the third Dos Equis) the story of the Cheapest Man in New York City. I told it to Rose.

"Seems El Cheapo needs dental treatment, but refuses to pay Park Avenue prices, even though that's where he lives. Eventually, he discovers the cheapest dentist in town. But before he goes in, he stops at a nearby store and queries the proprietor about the dentist. "Is he pain free?" he asks.

"Let me tell you a story, Mister," the storeowner answers. "I went to that dentist last summer for a new plate, and since it was so hot that day, I decided not to open the store after I'd left his office. Instead, I went to Central Park to cool off by the lake. When I got there, I rented a rowboat, but as I stepped in, I tripped and fell, impaling my crotch on one of the oarlocks. And for the first time that day,"—the proprietor leaned forward for the denouement—"my mouth didn't hurt!"

Rose didn't laugh. I, though, laughed so hard there were tears in my eyes.

When morning arrived, it brought with it two massive aches. Three Excedrins took care of one; the other, I knew, would need something much stronger and would, most surely, last a lot longer. And as if in tacit agreement, my rash decided to itch even more exquisitely than usual.

Over the next six days I worked at dredging up as much information about prostate cancer as I could. I studied the literature Mawn's office provided, pored over the few medical texts I had at home, nosed around mega-bookstores' medical sections, and browsed through texts at the library.

Whether laid out in simplistic form, or written in arcane medical jargon, it seemed to boil down to this: with age, prostates tend to enlarge, causing urinary problems, and in many cases (over 300,000 in '96) becoming cancerous. Available treatments are either operating, radiating, procrastinating or alternate medicating (hormonal therapy, nutritional miracle cures, the list is long).

Which of the treatment approaches to take depends on a sextet of variables: your age, physical condition, your prostate's condition, your doctor, your mate—and perhaps most important— your psyche.

How you feel about whether you and your aberrant prostate are willing to be chopped apart, burned by radiation, subjected to holistic nostrums, or just remain cliff-hanging, is the ultimate variable, the choice begrudgingly wrenched from somewhere inside your gut.

Even if you've boned up enough to duke out prostate cancer facts with a urologist, calculated the odds of survival (and the possible subsequent damage that can ensue), consulted every guru—from your Uncle Harry to your best-ever friend to your favorite religious advisor, and obtained second and possibly, third opinions—you've still got to dig around inside and choose—which choice you will question every day of your life until the post whatever-treatment-you-chose PSA test results come back. If your score is zero-point-practically-no-number-at-all, you've earned an A-plus with a gold star. A high score says you've failed and are awfully close to being kicked out of school. So much for the psyche variable.

Assuming all the prescribed prostate cancer tests are performed and analyzed correctly, and age and general health are within limits, the first three variables can be fixed and more easily ranked.

The mate variable is a lot harder to rate. It obviously depends on the myriad complexities that inform the relationship of two people who share their lives. I can only speak for mine. My mate's unequivocal love for me, her strength in support of me, and her fierce determination to protect and care for me in every way, especially during this unsettling time, rendered any variables in my mate rating moot. Rose scored a ten. Which leaves only the doctor variable to deal with.

Are your urologist's credentials impeccable? Hospital affiliations excellent? Success rate in the high nines? Malpractice suits few, if nonexistent? Do you like, respect, trust, feel comfortable with the doctor? For a high score, all questions should be answered with a decided "yes." Any other answers demand a second look at a second opinion.

I confess I didn't learn of the reference book, *"The Best Doctors In America,"* until two years past my prostate. But even if I had known of it, I still would have wanted personal references, some words of mouth. But as a newcomer to the Tampa Bay area, there weren't a lot of people in the medical fraternity I could turn to. The only two Florida doctors I knew were dentists. I had a high regard for them as dedicated professionals and human exemplars, and with no one else I could think to turn to, I turned to them.

David Dolgin, a paragon of periodontics, was the first one I corraled. A transplanted New Yorker, David and I shared a special background: we both attended Stuyvesant High School, Manhattan's prestigious science facility. We didn't know each other then, but that didn't matter; there's something about a school tie that indeed binds. The day David found out that we were both alumni of the same school, he stopped mid-exam, tore off his gloves, and went into his office, returning with an alumni bulletin, grinning as if he'd found a long lost brother.

When I asked what he knew about prostate cancer, he had to admit not much, but was acquainted with two doctors who'd been diagnosed with it. A year and a half after one doctor's surgery, David played golf with him, and he seemed to be in fine shape, winning the game by ten strokes.

The other doctor, who chose to watch and wait, wouldn't be playing golf anymore, since death (courtesy of an agressive type prostate cancer) has a way of putting a crimp in your game. Score one for surgery.

David did, though, know a urologist, someone he'd studied with at Columbia Medical School in New York City, but who was now practicing locally—a Doctor Bernard Hochberg. He was associated with St. Joseph's Hospital, same as Doctor Mawn. And St. Joe's, from what I'd been able to find out, had an excellent reputation. Points for the facility.

"Bernie's a top guy," David confided. "I haven't seen him in a while, but from everything I've heard, he's one of the best around. If you want a second opinion, he'd be a good choice."

David was sorry he couldn't be of more help, but even knowing the name of another urologist—especially one with a solid reputation—was more than enough assistance, since shopping for a doctor through the Yellow Pages was not my idea of how to go about getting an aspirin, let alone a second opinion.

After I'd thanked David and promised to keep him posted on

my progress, I drove over to my other dental connection—Sam Caranante. I'd grown to like and respect Sam during the nine months he'd worked on reclaiming my smile—lost over the years in an embarassing jumble of misshapen teeth. Smiling was an act I'd given up performing, so self-conscious was I about its unsightliness. (I still shudder at pictures of me taken with an assortment of famous movie and TV personalities who were acting as spokespersons in commercials I'd created. There I am, arms around some star, attempting a smile sans teeth, looking as if I were holding back a burp.)

I knew Sam would help me garner information with the same care and attention he'd put into reconstructing my mouth. After I'd told him what was up, Sam called an old school chum, now a local urologist and told him my story.

Sam's precis of his conversation with the doctor went like this: "If he's a young sixty-year old with Stage 2—operate. As for doctors, there are two A-list cutters in Tampa—Hochberg and Mawn. You can't go wrong with either of them."Points for surgery *and* doctors. And thank you, Sam.

I don't know if it was my age, my condition, or a little of both, but for the first time I realized I might, would, eventually die. As if with a snap of fingers, I had gone from the world's oldest living teenager to an infinitely finite man who was beginning to see what lay at the end of the road. And with that less-than-inspiring epiphany, came the need to connect with family and friends, share my current travail, maybe even pick up some important insights.

Besides, I had big stuff to talk about. These wouldn't be content-light, rambling conversations. After the hellos and the inevitable "How are you?," I would tell them, and after everyone caught their collective breaths, heated, incredibly invigorated hour-long discussions would most assuredly ensue.

My brother-in-law, Al Hampel, a renowned advertising executive, though sincerely concerned and fairly knowledgeable about the subject, couldn't add more to what I'd learned. But he did know a famed comedian-actor-director who, he informed me, had been operated on for prostate cancer a short while back and was now perfectly okay. Al shorthanded it like this: "You know Jerry. First thing he does is call DeBakey, best heart man in the world, who puts him onto the best urologist in the world, who, after checking him out, says operate. So Jerry has the operation." Al paused for emphasis. "And he was sixty-five at the time!"

That shored up the age variable quite a few notches.

Before I called Tommy and Sol, my longest-running friend-ships, I recalled how, over the years, we cheered each other's achievements. Unfortunately, I had now arrived at a place no one wanted to go, let alone cheer about. A less ignominious first would have been preferable, but when you've shared even the smallest tidbits since high school, every first counts. A guy thing, obviously.

If nothing else, we'd have livelier conversations than we'd had in a long time. As contemporaries, they would want to, and had to, know about this turn of events, since there, but for the grace of God, genes and good luck, it could befall them as well. I foresaw long distance charges on both sides rivaling the national debt.

Sol's offering, over and above his love and good wishes, was a vitamin regimen to be followed from now till forever, or at least until the crisis was past. It was a long list which I vowed to follow to the letter. Naturally, Sol wanted to know if I had considered any alternate medical approaches, but mercifully didn't pursue the subject after I said I had, and had dismissed them. I'm sure he felt I wasn't exploring enough alternate venues (living in Southern California for over thirty years will do that to you), but in his heart of hearts was lighting candles for my recovery, praying that I was doing the right thing. I could feel him hugging me all the way from Los Angeles.

Sol also pushed me to train for this event.

Every other day, after a rigorous warmup routine, I did three sets of crunchies, leg raises and pushups—after which I went out for a three mile power walk, finishing with a seven flight climb to my condo aerie. I was going to be in good shape for whatever was to come even if it killed me.

Tommy, in an earlier life, must have been the guy Moses first handed the tablets off to. He was our Solon, our very own F. Lee Bailey, the one we turned to for legal counsel, brilliant, world-class conversation, and marvelous, mischievous wit. Even during his grilling me to ascertain that I had, and was, asking the right questions and checking out the situation from every angle, Tommy was able to make me laugh. Time and again, as chagrined and disheartened by this crummy life development as we both were, Tommy would send my spirits soaring with some sweet humor to offset the bitterness of the situation, like the expresso he introduced me to a hundred years ago when the world was a lot younger. If laughter is medicine, as many claim, Tommy was one of my most important prescriptions. His words were balm. And his ears were a stethoscope, listening to the tenor of my voice as carefully as he listened to the voices of the many world-famous singers he produced songs and albums for—outstanding creative efforts which earned him a wallful of gold and platinum records and a solid financial future.

Tommy never missed a note. He could hear when I was scared, or being evasive, or just plain bullshitting, though I forever tried to bluff him out by using my "What! Me worry?" voice. But he always heard between the lines, knew when I was off-key, when my pitch wasn't perfect. He was my sometimes twice daily dose of reality and wonderful humor, which never failed to knock me out, and in so doing, took me, if only for a moment, out of myself, soaring high above my cares, out of harm's way. I always felt Tommy's arm around me, squeezing a shot of courage into my shoulder as if he were around the corner, not a continent away in San Francisco. I don't think I ever felt closer.

The smartest woman I know, other than Rose, is Shellie. Her quick, inquisitive mind, zany sense of humor, daring leaps of faith, extraordinary ability to verbalize and most of all, that we share a lifetime in and out of the advertising business make her an A-list best friend. Her strength and pluck constantly leave me in awe: she's the only one I know who's done EST twice; the only one I know who's had the balls to actually walk on hot coals as if she were a card-carrying voodoo fellow traveler; the only person I know who, in spite of more than a dozen debilitating years, has managed to survive, learn, grow and prosper.

It was only natural that once I told Shellie the latest news of my life, she would go into high holistic gear and sound me out about alternate paths to a cure. Had I, she asked, looked into homeopathy, meditation, acupuncture, coffee enemas or the latest therapy panacea of the moment—visualization?

Shellie meant well, but I had to balk at visualization. *Let's see, Shel. I visualize my prostate. Then I visualize the cancer in my prostate. Then I visualize it shrinking. And then what? Visualize myself dying!? Shellie—a mind meld with Spock makes more scientific sense than that!*

I didn't need to apologize. Shellie understood my edginess, felt my pain and sent me her best karma to help me in the arduous trek I was about to embark on. She also sent me a book on some breakthrough miracle cancer cures she had discovered at her favorite health food store. These were Shellie's good wishes for my survival, and though I didn't take them all in, I cherished them nonetheless.

Mel and I started out in the advertising business together and have been the best of friends ever since. Sales promotion was his forte. The only Jewish leprechaun in existence, Mel could charm someone into buying a rock, having convinced them it was gold. He could also revert to his Brooklyn cum Astoria roots when called for. This was one of those times. No reminiscing about the fact that we both had to work in our fathers' candy stores even while attending college. No politically incorrect jokes. No bitching about the "business" going to hell in a handbasket. Hearing I had prostate cancer made Melvin Brian Klein angry. He'd recently lost two friends to the disease, and that I was now threatened by it only served to get his Irish up.

"Tell me you've got the best goddamned doctor you can get or I'll drag your ass up here!" Up here, naturally, meant the Big Apple. Mel knows for a fact that anything outside of New York City doesn't count; that Manhattan has the best of everything, is the center of the world—no, the universe—and is the only place on earth to go to save your bacon.

He wouldn't let up on me until I convinced him that I was, indeed, exploring every option, getting second opinions, the whole schmear. I had to explain my every move, but no gory details, please. The least mention of a hypodermic, let alone a specific procedure gave Mel the willies. It was too close; it could be him. I understood.

He called every day for an update, finishing each conversation with, "You're gonna be okay!"—his prayer, odds-on bet and threat all in one, his way of lighting candles. I had to be okay or he'd kick my ass.

Of course, a host of other friends and business associates were on my "must tell" list—yet, of all these people, none knew a lot about prostate cancer except that it was something dire to contemplate, nor—other than my brother-in-law and my pal Mel—knew anyone who had had it and survived. Which cut off a potential source of networking for possible insights and important first hand feedback. But to a person, they challenged my research, my assumptions, and my fears, desperately hoping I was making sense and, more important, the right decisions. Granted, they were not all wholeheartedly in favor of my leaning to the side of traditional medicine, but they were, nevertheless, in my corner.

Even though it's not listed in the pharmacoepia of curing potions, loving support, I learned, can be as important as medicine.

My grownup daughter, Lori Joy, became hysterical when I told her what was up. But after I dried her tears with an inspired, rosy picture of the outlook, even though she didn't buy the whole story (no fool, she), she held onto it throughout the ordeal. So did I. Daddy's girl, in forcing me to examine the up side of the situation—something I'd not yet been able to do—had me considering that the glass might, indeed, be half full.

My son, David, took in the grim news thoughtfully, gently questioning me about the choices, the ramifications of each, the doctor's pedigree, the hospital's "kill ratio" (blame his father's sense of humor), the works. This moon child showed how much of a man he was during this ugly business.

Besides, I wasn't going to die; my children wouldn't allow it.

Next to Rose, my friends and family were the rocks I clung to as my purchase on the world gave new meaning to the expression "holding on by your fingertips."

Chapter 3

Acceptance Prerequisites

My desk calendar began to look like it used to when I was a Creative Director, but instead of meetings with writers, art directors, producers, directors, casting agents, composers and suits of every stripe, it was appointments with doctors, hospitals and laboratories. Prostate cancer was not only overtaking my body, it had invaded my life.

All I could do was think, talk and read about it. All-consuming doesn't come close to describing the condition.

Adenocarcinoma not only takes over your gland, it takes over your mind, even when you're asleep. Before I had my bone and CAT scans, I dreamt a whopper.

I am walking down the hospital-width halls of a broadcasting empire of which, for some strange reason, I am the Executive Producer. It is the newly-spawned Medical Network (MNC) which programs everything and anything medical twenty-four hours a day.

Now I'm sitting in a darkened screening room, staring at a wallful of TV screens, making omnipotent programming decisions.

"Mark, don't forget to highlight the call-in feature for those dolts who don't even know they have a bloody prostate—or even where it is! (I somehow know that all assistant producers are named Mark.)

It appears I'm talking about one of the early morning features—"Dear Doctor," a telephone, write-in, fax-in, E-mail-in, question and answer show, hosted by a hirsute Doctor Tom.

The first question the announcer reads has a familiar ring.

"Dear Doctor, My husband's been told he has prostate cancer. He's 61 years of age, in good health, except for his skin rash. What would you recommend—radiation or a radical prostatectomy? Sincerely, Missus R.G., St. Petersburg."

The host answers: "Mrs. G., until we know the results of your hubby's CAT and bone scans, we can't give you a definitive answer at the moment. But call us when you find out what they are, and we'll chat about it then. Okay?"

I hear myself saying: "Mark, whatever you do, don't let Mawn lose the white beard! It gives him a certain gravitas this show needs! This sick market is huge! Let's take a meeting and kick around the numbers on that rerun deal with the "Dr. Kildare" syndicators. Find out if they ever did an episode on prostate cancer."

I am about to call Ted Turner to tell him I cannot do lunch when my bladder signals me awake.

I didn't need a Freudian analyst to explain this transparent production. The hidden agenda didn't take much to analyze, either. I was obviously dreaming I could script the answer. I guess I'll have to review the tape again, not just the opening credits and the first few minutes of the show. Maybe another night.

To be at St. Joe's for my CAT and bone scan at a quarter to seven in the morning means I have to be up by 4:30 AM, a dark beginning to this April 5th Monday.

The drive to Tampa invigorates me. I get to watch the sunrise as it dawns over Tampa Bay, painting color into the fading night so intensely, it stirs me as it awakens Hillsborough County. I also get to redline my MR2 up to six grand, blowing unwanted carbon off the plugs, exercising the valves, and scaring myself silly while speeding into the day.

I arrive at the hospital exhilarated and as ready as one can be for whatever assorted discomforts today's tests may bring. (My rectum still winces at the thought of the dildo from hell they euphemistically call an ultra-sound probe.) And even though I understand that these tests are necessary in ruling out the possible metastasis of the prostate cancer, knowing isn't quite sufficient to dispel the queasiness.

St. Joe's reception area is spacious, all glass and soft morning light, and at 6:45 AM, as crowded as a railroad station at rush hour. A wave of people surge toward the reception desk, eager to check in and begin their journey back to health. The remainder fill the closely-set chairs, grimly waiting for a signal that their train is about to get on track.

I join the throng at the Nurse's Admitting Station, sign in and find a seat amongst the travelers As protection from year-old *People* magazines, and to prevent myself from staring at the innumerable wheel chairs, crutch collections and bandaged limbs that surround me, I keep my eyes fixed on the *Herald Tribune* crossword puzzle book I'd brought along to pass the time and spare me from thinking of anything but a word for a word I've never heard of to begin with. Besides, I am too tan, altogether too healthy to be here. I feel out of place and somehow embarrassed.

Forget eye contact; like my fellow passengers, I seek protection in anonymity. Head down, I try to remain faceless. If no one sees me then I'm not here; fantasy *mishegas* of the first order. Anxiety will do that to you every time.

After only just beginning the first puzzle, my name is called. At the reception desk, I'm asked to have a seat and told to drink—within fifteen minutes—a quart of an artificially-flavored-with-pine-apple-to keep-you-from-puking liquid that makes the intestines visible for the pelvic C/T scan.

"We keep it chilled so it won't be so bad," the too perky nurse informs me. She also warns that it might upset my stomach on its way to the site, and that I had to wait a few hours.

The hours pass quickly enough—in the men's room. From the moment I finish my cocktail, I begin to receive telegraph messages from my lower intestines, and am consigned to quick-trotting across the rotunda all morning, feeling that by my fifth dash for the toilets, I am the center of attention. *Poor man. What could be wrong! Maybe he's one of those pervs who hang out in men's toilets! Probably messed his pants!*

The C/T scan, which, thankfully, only has to peruse my pelvic area, saves me from having to go all the way inside the tunnel-like device. I'm not claustrophobic, but if I can avoid being rolled inside a small cave, thank you very much.

The only hitch in the procedure is that the technician can't find—after four unsuccessful stabs—a vein to inject the dye into. (The dye clearly delineates the kidneys, liver and lymph nodes so it can be determined whether or not the tumor has spread beyond the prostate into any of these adjacent tissues.)

He is nervous, embarrassed and, I sense, gay. And each time he misses the mark, he half-pats, half-squeezes my shoulder. Nothing erotic, solely a human touch, his hand saying, "I'm sorry I'm not better at this. I know how uncomfortable it is." His touch is somehow comforting, because someone in this tangle of ominous-looking contraptions, someone acknowledges my existence as a warm body, not just a control number on a chart. It comes to me that perhaps belief in the laying on of hands is not without merit. If I were a medicine man, I'm convinced that touch, or "non-allopathic palliatives," as alternate medicine calls it, would be one of my most-prescribed pain relievers.

After a last abortive attempt to skewer a vein, the technician admits defeat and calls in a senior nurse to do the honors. I squeeze his forearm to tell him it's okay, I understand.

The bone scan went much better. Three hours after the injection of a radioactive tracer, I was scanned by a device that outlined my skeleton, looking for hot spots that would show up if the cancer had spread to bone.

It is almost noon by the time I get into my car for the drive home. The day has become overcast, mirroring my mood. The tests, with their disconcerting clank and whir, the "green apple quicks" from the pineapple puke juice, the track marks on my arm, and my apprehension about what I will hear on Friday (my next appointment with Doctor Mawn), have sapped my energy, and it takes all my concentration to steer the car.

Friday, though only three days after the bone and CAT scans, seemed to take an eternity to arrive. Blame it on clockwatching. Checking the time every few minutes is guaranteed to slow things down, never letting anything come to a boil. Staring at the clock, waiting for the countdown is like willing time to stand still, and if you wish hard enough, maybe Friday won't come after all, and you won't have to find out that the time bomb ticking inside you has already exploded.

Illness, I discovered, warps your perception of time, first dragging, now fleeting, as if you were stranded somewhere in a Dali landscape, your normal perceptions distorted. Case in point: once Friday did arrive, it seemed to come too quickly, and we found ourselves sitting opposite Tom Mawn, wondering where the time went.

"Good news, guys." Tom is beaming. "You're clean! The C/ T scan *and* the bone scan show no signs of the cancer having escaped from the prostate. Looks like it's self-contained."

As if rehearsed, Rose and I both exhale loudly and mock collapse in relief. Another hurdle overcome.

"Have you come to any decision, yet?" Tom asks, offering to review the treatment options. I wave the offer off. He has to move things along. Though it's late afternoon, his waiting room is crowded. How many men today, I wonder, will he not have good news for.

"We're close to it, Tom. But I still have to see the radiotherapist and hear what he has to say."

"Yes, that's important. But I also want to schedule you for an IVP. It's an X-ray of your urinary tract to check for any obstructions or tumors in the kidneys, bladder or ureter. It's a bit redundant, and a lot of doctors don't call for it once the C/T is negative, but I like to double check."

I am too elated at having a clean bill of health to allow the question "double check what?" to surface and spook me. I didn't crap out today and wanted nothing to spoil it.

Tom again offers to review the treatment options, but I decline on the grounds that I'm on option overload and have to give it a rest for awhile.

In the parking lot, Rose and I high five it and then hug each other hard.

Over our first Margarita at Rio Bravo, we fumble to come up with an appropriate toast, settling for "Thank God it's Friday!," laughing some of our angst away, happy for the moment.

DAYBOOK ENTRY: 4/8/94

Patient: Bert Gottlieb

Reason for Visit: Discuss results of imaging tests and review treatment options.

Followup: Intravenous Pyelogram. (CT scan was essentially normal save for some fullness of the distal left ureter, this of undetermined clinical significance, but bears looking into.)

Post Visit Thoughts & Observations: This was the first good news I could deliver to the Gottliebs—that both the bone and pelvic CT scan were negative for evidence of distant spread. It was also the time to review the current medical status of prostate cancer in general, and Bert's problem specifically.

Now that the brain-numbing pronouncement of the C-word had been uttered, and he and his family have had time to recover from the shock of hearing it, there still remained the task of dealing with it. And while some of the emotional heat generated by the bad news will have dissipated, permitting a cooler, more sober appraisal of the situation, it is still an emotion-laden ordeal for most patients.

In my experience, and that of my colleagues, this visit is perhaps the most important one, because in most cases, eighty-five percent of the decision process will occur at this meeting, and it should proceed as cooly and rationally as possible.

The Gottliebs had done their homework since I'd last seen them, processed the information I'd provided, as well as what they'd learned on their own, narrowed down their options, and wanted nothing more than to celebrate their joy (and mine) that the tumor appeared contained within the prostate.

On Wednesday, the thirteenth of April, I report to St. Joe's at the most reasonable hour of 9:30 AM for this kidney test.

Next to the bone scan with its noxious preparations, the IVP is cake. Even the warning by Doctor Mandelblatt that once the dye enters the blood stream it may cause a burning feeling coursing throughout the body—a normal response in many patients, one that would soon pass—doesn't shake me. What's a temporary temperature compared to the runs, or your arm being used as a dart board! Granted, I was on red alert, awaiting the onslaught of the heat, but it never came. I admit there was a slight warming trend, but it was so momentary and mild, had the affable doctor omitted his warning, it might have passed unnoticed, or if felt, been interpreted as a hot flash of some sort, a reaction to the strange and chilly surroundings.

During the week before I was to meet with Doctor John West at the Woods Radiation Center for the radiation consultation, I called Doctor Hochberg's office to set up an appointment for a second opinion, only to learn that he was on vacation and wouldn't be back for two weeks.

In a way, I was glad. Somehow, stupidly many will say, I felt that going for a second opinion was like cheating on your doctor—as if you didn't respect his knowledge and experience, his judgment, the test results; that you didn't trust him because maybe, just maybe, his interests weren't in *your* best interests.

In spite of my urologist having urged me to seek a second opinion—out of, I'm sure, utter confidence that *his* opinion would be held up, *and* to relieve me of any second thoughts I might have had—I was not pleased at the prospect because I *did* trust him. I felt there was a bond between us that transcended the doctor-patient relationship—a bond between two men. Tom was one of the few men I'd met over all my years that I wouldn't be afraid to be in a foxhole with. So confident was I that he'd do everything to protect my back (not to mention other important parts), that I'd have bet my life on it, irrational a thought as that was.

With that in mind, a second opinion was put on the shelf.

On the morning of April 18th, I drive to the Woods Radiation Center and find it easily, even though it's only 8:45, a tick too early for me to function at peak. Luckily, St. Joe's is next door, so I don't have to strain my direction-challenged brain in a search for a low-slung building in Tampa, a city that blossoms with low-slung buildings.

Doctor West seems pleasant and capable as he explains the process involved in external-beam radiation therapy, that they do a special C/T scan for treatment planning, and use other advanced guidance systems to pinpoint the target they're aiming at, that the treatment is five times a week for around eight weeks, and that after the third week or so, some patients experience stomach distress, which usually clears up once the treatment is over. Also, that the success rate of this therapy is ninety-five percent.

When I ask him whether the fact that I have diverticulosis

should be of concern, considering that the diverticula were, it seemed to me, in the line of fire, he says, "We try our best to avoid those areas."

Having been in advertising most of my working life, "try" was the wrong word to use with me. "Try," along with "may" and "can" are the ultimate weasel words, the legal way around the inability to make a flat-out claim. To the uninitiated, these hedges are usually never noticed. If anything, they sometimes strengthen the claim. *This cream* can *help you have a more beautiful skin! This vitamin* may *be just what the doctor ordered! We'll* try *our best to avoid those areas! And the check* is *in the mail!*

What I wanted to hear, and didn't, was, "We *will* avoid those areas!" So I turned a deaf ear to external-beam radiation. It didn't pass my truth-in-advertising test.

The radioactive seed implantation discussion takes about as long as how to figure out the pronunciation of interstitial brachytherapy, the formal name for the seeding process.

It is a good, if general, overview. But what isn't mentioned are the high odds of impotency, or even the low odds of diarrhea, painful bowel movements, rectal bleeding, skin eruptions (as if my current ones weren't enough), urinary complications, excessive tiredness and loss of energy, or any other collateral damage that might ensue. And that it can take from three weeks to three months—or even longer in some cases—after the first session for the symptoms to disappear. Nor does he offer the information, until I ask him, that with seeding, there are no longer-term tracking statistics than five years. And in neither case, does he inform me that surgery is not an option if the recipient is one of the unlucky five percent, or if his cancer recurs (which it does in thirty to ninety percent of patients, according to *The Reader's Digest*, one of the least hysterical voices on issues of this sort). He also doesn't mention that radiation therapy is an ideal option for an older person, but not for a man like me, who has the potential to live many more years. The little sins of omission.

To his credit, Doctor West doesn't lean hard on either of the approaches. His presentation is straightforward, rather laidback, a here-they-are, take-your-pick approach. *If, for whatever reason, you can't countenance having your prostate sliced out by a knife, preferring it to be burned out instead, there's external-beam therapy. And if two months or so of treatment seems too long, we can also seed your prostate and have you out in a day. Your choice.*

Before I leave, he wishes me well, and I tell him I'll have to think about everything he's told me before I make my mind up, which, of course, he understands. The truth is, I'd decided against radiation treatments even before we said goodbye.

DAYBOOK ENTRY: 4/18/94

Patient: BG

Call to Dr. West: Discussed treatment options and the fact that patient has not yet made up his mind. However, if he elects to undergo external beam radiation, I would recommend Lupron or, better yet, Proscar be prescribed prior to the procedure to shrink the prostate, which appears too large at this point to consider transperineal ultrasonically-guided seed insertion.

Wednesday is a Doctor Mawn day, the day we should have some answer for him as to which road we've chosen to take, which makes Tuesday, today, decision day.

Unlike a business, where decisions are made after hour-long discussions of issues, a vote, and then lunch, decision-making in a marriage is far less structured, with mini-meetings covering all the necessary topics taken over the course of a day, and a vote taken somewhere between brushing teeth and crawling into bed to watch the news.

7:00 AM, over tea—chamomile for Rose, black currant for me—the first of the mini-meetings.

I kick things off. "I'll never forget the sound of Doctor Dominguez's voice when he told me about my PSA doubling like that from the year before."

"He did send you to a good urologist," Rose adds.

"Yeah, let the good urologist deliver the good news."

"At least your Gleason grade is good, and the staging okay, so the sucker seems to be self-contained."

"Is "sucker" really a medical term?"

Suddenly sober, Rose asks, "The tests were done right, weren't they?"

I'd thought about that, but aside from the petty discomforts, the actual tests were performed with total concentration; every inch of me measured, focused on and monitored as if I were the only body in the world.

"If any of the tests got screwed up, or if there was something iffy about the results, they'd have had me back in a New York minute. You want another cup of tea?"

12:30 PM, and mini-meeting two starts while I'm mincing onion and celery for the tuna fish, and Rose is gathering the mayo, lemon and dill weed.

"Did you ever call Doctor . . . the one David Dolgin told you about . . . for a second opinion?"

"Doctor Hochberg. Yes, I did, beginning of last week. He was on vacation and wouldn't be back till tomorrow."

Rose hands me the mayo jar. "Not too much," she cautions.

"Besides, what's he gonna tell me? That I *don't* have prostate cancer? That the tests are invalid? That Tom *didn't* feel a nodule? That the biopsy, the Gleason score, the staging were invalid? That I should go home and forget about it?"

"I like the last part."

"Me, too. You want the tuna on crackers or toast?"

7:00 PM, the third mini-meeting is in session over black rum and OJ for Rose, two fingers of single malt for me, this, while I deftly devein the shrimp I'm going to scampify for our dinner.

"Whaddya think?" I ask, no subject needed.

Rose takes a manicured shrimp from me and lays it thoughtfully on a plate.

"You're too young for watchful wondering," she says.

"*Waiting.* Watchful *waiting.*"

"Too young to be wondering, anyway."

Rose slaps a shrimp crosswise over the first one she'd put on the plate. "I hear there's a man, somewhere in Asia," I say, putting alternate medicine on the table, "who can literally reach inside you and pluck out the offending organ, gland, cancer, whatever. And he doesn't leave a hole! I mean, there's no bleeding! They've got it on film. *Mondo Something-Or-Other.*

In response, Rose deftly palms a shrimp, then makes believe she's pulling it out of my lower stomach. "Like this, you mean?"

"Jest if you will, but there's an old lady in Taipei who'd be delighted to show you her gall bladder . . . with *no* scar."

"What should we have with the shrimp—linguini or cappellini?"

"How about chelation therapy?"

"*What* kind of therapy?"

"Shellie sent me a monograph on it. It's a natural roto-rooter for the blood. They dose you with EDTA, which is supposed to bind with all the dreck in your system, eventually flushing it all out in your urine."

"Only?"

"Only that the first page is full of classic hedge words—may, can, helps to, could, should—but so well-written it almost sounds believable."

"The art of the copywriter personified." Rose points a finger at me.

"I never lied."

"You hedged."

"Sometimes. Only when it was trivial. You want grated cheese?"

8:00 PM. In between slurping up linguini and watching a rerun of *Seinfeld*, the next to last mini-discussion ensues.

I begin with a flourish. "To radiate . . . or *not* to radiate? That *is* the question." Rose picks it up. "Whether 'tis nobler in the mind of man to suffer the slings and arrows of his outrageous ass being assaulted from the outside . . . or from the inside?"

"Forget the question," I answer.

"I'm going into the kitchen. Do you want more shrimp?"

11:00 PM. The final choice is debated and voted on by both parties, while the local weather tease calls for a cloudy tomorrow.

"Well?" No subject needed again.

"Out." Rose's vote.

"There's always the chance of incontinence and or impotence."

"We could figure out a way," Rose offers mischievously.

"Seriously, what if . . . "

"What if I told you I loved you?"

"You didn't answer the question."

"Yes, I did."

"They take out the seminal vesicles, you know."

"That doesn't take out the fun!"

"I hope not . . . but what if I'm left leaking, having to wear diapers, like a . . . " I couldn't bring myself to say the word baby.

"It won't happen."

"From your mouth to Godzilla's ears!"

"And if it *does* happen we'll deal with it."

"So it's *out, out damned prostate!*"

"I thought Lady Macbeth had that line."

"Okay. *Out.*"

"Look! Steven Wright's one of Leno's guests!"

"You'll be asleep before they drag him out. Let's watch a *DS9* rerun, instead."

"Go to sleep."

"Jesus, Rose."

"I know."

Why do people say "let me sleep on this " before making a decision, when nighttime is when decisions are made? In the dark of your bed, you'll chew over every factor, examining each detail from every angle, whether you and a couple of Tylenol PMs want to sleep or not.

I can still recall the first (and only) time I had to give the axe to someone. I was the newly-hired Creative Director of an umpteen million-dollar advertising agency, and one of my inherited staff was not producing, nor even trying to. His only creative effort seemed to be avoiding me.

After a couple of lectures cum dutch uncle talks, plus months of rope, he still wasn't working out; if anything, he got worse. I knew I had to let him go. It wasn't fair to the other copywriters who had to shoulder his work. Nor to him, for that matter.

When, on the rare occasion I'd manage to catch a glimpse of him, he looked terrible: haunted, angry, mega-fucked up. It was time. Yet it took all night to examine all the reasons for letting him go. Wide-awake, I questioned every motive. Was I, the new top gun of the creative department, perhaps demonstrating that I was no one's pushover? Or was I merely flexing corporate muscle to show the suits I could make the tough decisions? And I hated the way he dressed. Could I really be that petty? From the inspired to the ridiculous, my brain wouldn't rest until it was satisfied that the decision was well and fairly made.

He took the news far worse than I had expected, and was

packed up and out of the office before the day was over, without even a goodbye to people he'd known for years.

Occasionally, I'd ask other staffers if they'd heard from him. They said they'd called him a few times, but he wasn't very talkative and never called back. I saw him hanging in the despair of his apartment; that I had been the one who kicked the chair away.

Then one day, a year later, he bounded into my office, hugged me as if I were a long lost amigo, and thanked me no end for having "pushed him out of the nest."

After a year of blaming, sucking his thumb and pondering what had happened, he concluded that I was right to have canned him. And with this acceptance, came permission to climb the dozen steps needed to fly on his own. After which pop therapy, he'd polished up his portfolio, registered with a trendy body snatcher and landed a new position for more money than he'd been making before, and let's do lunch sometime.

It was worth losing a night's sleep.

But once you've decided things, it would seem your mind would heed the "lights out" caution and turn itself off. Not this night, the night before the day I have to choose behind which door the tiger isn't. Even though the vote was taken and the choice inevitable, as Rose gently snores beside me, my head begins to gnaw on what has been gone over ad nauseum since the inception of my prostate cancer worries. No question is left unturned as I watch the television screen, seeing and hearing nothing but a chorus of inner scolds. Their catechism is not only strict, they demand true faith; one must believe in every answer.

On top of the universal doubts they raise, a host of talmudic "what if's" are thrown in to enliven things. The one I keep stumbling over is: "What if the second opinion (which you didn't get!) was that you didn't have to be operated on?" "That's ridiculous!" I answer each time, which, while true, doesn't quite suffice and continues to nag—a toothache in my conscience. If guilt could be converted to energy, OPEC would have to give their oil away.

To divert my mind from its inquisition, I turn the volume up on *The Philadelphia Story*. A too-young Cary Grant, Katharine Hepburn, Jimmy Stewart, and a delicious script captivates me, but before I can find out who Kate is going to marry, I fall into a fretful sleep.

When I awake, I recollect a dream fragment: my doctor is Grant, Hepburn his nurse and Stewart the surgeon. Taking off his surgical mask, Stewart leans over me and says: "Bert, we ah . . . got it out but you won't be playing the ah . . . piano anymore." I am mildly convinced, as I pull on a robe, that inside me dwells a madman, made even crazier by its, my, our condition—and like a vampire, is sucking my brains out while I sleep. "What if," the talmudic voice persists as I stumble into the bathroom, "What if it were true? About the piano playing, that is?"

Since our appointment with Doctor Mawn isn't until mid-afternoon, there's plenty of time to exorcise the sleep demons before the real me has to face up to the day.

As I sign in at the front desk, I notice that Mawn's waiting room is not as crowded as usual—just two ghostly couples staring dispiritedly into some inner space. Will we, I wonder, soon look like them? Inside, I know we are as pale and diminished as the most dejected of souls sitting around us. But will our tans fade, the color drain from our lives as it seems to have from theirs? I wish I could grab Rose by the arm and run with her into the daylight.

"Mister Gottlieb?" Annette opens the door and beckons me in for the obligatory urine specimen.

I'd found, well before learning I had prostate cancer and my subsequent reading about it, that when the stream is reluctant to start, squeezing hard is not the answer. Some half-recalled high school physics theory about water needing air to pour freely out of a container tells me not to strain, but rather to relax and wait, and the liquid eventually will flow out. (If it doesn't, a reaming out of the urethra becomes a distinct possibility.)

My cram course in male urological problems has also taught me that working your bladder by straining (albeit instinctively) to force the urine out, is like working any set of muscles: they get built up, and the more muscle in the walls of the bladder, the less room for urine. Thus the need to urinate more often.

So I concentrate on relaxing and let nature take its (snail-like, by now) course. When I'm finished, we're directed to the doctor's office.

After we're seated, Tom asks us right off whether we've thought about our choices and come to any conclusions.

I stare at the floor, then at Rose—a last minute check that we're in synch— "I . . . we've . . . I think we've decided to . . . to go ahead with the radical."

"You're doing the right thing," Tom says.

"We hope so," Rose and I say at the same time, as if rehearsed—which rates a chuckle and allows us to let out our breath.

"Let me tell you about the procedure, then," Tom says, sensing the shift.

"The operation takes about four or so hours. I recommend the epidural anaesthetic. It's the best way to go for pain control. Once we're in, the first thing we do is remove the lymph glands and send them to pathology to make sure they're clean."

"What do you do while you're waiting—play cards on my chest?" A futile attempt to lighten my mood which, despite outward appearances, is beginning to head downhill rapidly as I recall reading that if lymph glands are found to be tainted, they stop the procedure, close you up and pretty much kiss your ass goodbye.

"Y'know, I never thought of that," Tom answers. "Maybe I'll bring a deck of cards with me when I *do* you," he says with a twinkle in his eye, but then quickly adds, as if to assure us he's only kidding, "We're kept pretty busy in the OR."

The fact that Tom feels he has to assure us he is merely jesting makes me like him even more. Seriousness in defense of one's professionalism, especially when it's not necessary is, indeed, a fetching quality.

"Your hospital stay will be about five days—depends on you and how everything goes. First couple of days you'll be in intensive care. Then we get you to a room. There'll be a couple of drains coming out of you to get rid of any unwanted blood and clots. You'll be on an IV dripping antibiotics into you to prevent any post-operative infections. And, of course, you'll be catheterized—not only during the hospital stay—but for three weeks afterward. Saves your system from having to work while it's busy working to heal."

My rash is itching so badly, I have all to do from jumping up, dropping my pants and tearing at my skin.

"I want you to give blood, too," Tom says.

"Isn't that what blood banks are for?" I ask, my voice unexpectedly leaping into a falsetto.

"Your blood likes you. If we're going to need blood—and we might—I want it to be the best blood—and that's yours. Okay?"

It is not okay, but I begrudgingly agree.

I remembered the first (and last) time I agreed to give blood. It was over 35 years ago. I was a young copywriter at a prestigious ad agency and everybody was giving blood, so why not. When it came time to go in, even though I tried to put on a face, the doctor saw how scared I was and washed me out before I had to look at a needle. I even recalled him muttering something about my looking as if I were coming down with a cold and therefore, shouldn't be donating; a gentle letting down, and a good excuse for my co-workers.

"How many pints?" Rose asks before I return from my reverie.

"Five," Tom answers. "And here's a prescription for an iron supplement your blood will begin to need." He tears the script off the pad and hands it to me. "Any other questions?" he asks as if he had all the time in the world.

I know I have a hundred questions, but none of them are available at the moment. I can't think for the itching.

I look to Rose for help.

"You've done this operation before?" Rose asks. A whimsical challenge.

Tom grins. "Once or twice. I've lost count."

"And *you'll* be doing it?" My feisty prosecutor is on the case.

"Of course!" Tom answers as if that were not a question.

"And your success rate is ninety-five percent?"

Tom nods yes.

A long pause. "And you'll wash your hands good?" Laughs all around.

As Tom walks us out, he hugs Rose's shoulder. "It's going to be fine, Rose," he assures her, not selling, merely squeezing in a shot of confidence. "We'll talk again. Before the operation, I'll answer any questions you have. Now I'm going to put you in the hands of the person who really runs this operation."

Cindy is as proficient an office administrator as Tom said she would be. She makes a molehill out of the mountain of paperwork to be gone over. The hardest part of the process is deciding on a date for the operation. Even though I understand there is no rush, that the slow-grow nature of this type of carcinoma allows me as much time as I need to make up my mind, I want this leg of the journey to be behind me. I know where I'm headed. I just want to know when I get there. I need to be rid of the angst that pervades my life. I also need a lucky number.

When Cindy informs me that the doctor will be on vacation

the first two weeks in June, but has hospital duty the last weekend in May, and that Friday is one of his operating days, I okay Friday, May 27th for the big event, numerology be damned.

As she calmy pencils me in on her calendar, considering what it took to get to this moment, I half expect fireworks. *How about a highlighter, Cindy? A colored pen? A red pencil?* I have just committed myself to Chapter Two of this horror story, and more should be made of it than an armful of instructions, telephone numbers and when and where to report. I need trumpets to drown out the whiny voice that continues to ask "What if . . . ?"

I want to be deaf to my doubts. The only words I need to hear are from a server asking if I want another Margarita.

DAYBOOK ENTRY: 4/20/94

Patient: BG
Reason for Visit: Conference to discuss patient's decision.
Recap: Bert has decided, albeit reluctantly and begrudgingly, to proceed with a radical retropubic prostatectomy, which he understands will be done in conjunction with a laparoscopic pelvic lymphadenectomy to ensure there is no cancer in the lymph nodes before proceeding with the surgery.
Post Visit Thoughts & Observations: His urge to "get it out" is, as with so many patients, exceedingly strong, and a normal, all too human need for tangible proof that the cancer has been removed. And yet, as I've explained, there are no absolutes. Even with the tumorous gland removed, an unseen, unexcised cell lurking in his system could begin the process again. Which is why Bert will be checked, with his PSA level tested, every six months for ten or more years, when statistically it will be safe to say—if his PSA results remain consistently in the zero point low number range during that time—he's out of the woods.

Reviewed, with a bit more detail, the operational outlines, reiterated the post-operative possibilities regarding incontinence and erectile disfunction, and instructed patient to start autologous blood donations (5 in total), and begin taking Mol-Iron supplements (l tab tid).

The decision to proceed with a radical prostatectomy is fraught with doubt and as emotionally upheaving as the months preceding the decision. It is perhaps one of the most difficult choices anyone has to face. And in spite of only guessing at what inner turmoil they've gone through to arrive at their decision, Bert and Rose seem to have faced it squarely and intelligently, and I'm confident they will cope well in spite of the trying times ahead of them.

Rose and I make love that night more as an act of healing than a romantic romp. Yet even after relief has suffused us with peace, we still sleep fitfully. It's a wonder we can sleep at all.

* * *

Chapter 4

Background Investigation

Wednesday, April twenty-seventh. I am late for my 1:30 PM appointment at the blood donor facility located within St. Joe's. I'm never late. Being on time is a compulsion. Only once did I ever miss a plane—by this much. The image of my clients waving to me from the windows of the plane as I stand on the tarmac, sweating like a pig and panting from a run from another terminal, has never left me. I always add a bumper just in case there's heavy traffic or an earthquake. Better to fiddle with a puzzle waiting your turn, than feel the acid eating at your innards while you're gridlocked.

Today, though, I drag my heels, leave no room for error, and wind up chewing on a Maalox tab as I reluctantly climb the stairs to the collection site.

The Southwest Florida Blood Bank is brightly lit, with a small reception area, diminutive cubicles on the side, and a large, arena-like main section with four bed-couches per side, facing each other. *The better to see each drainee draining?*

At the cramped reception desk, I fill out a questionnaire, sign a consent release, but am stumped by a form entitled "Autologous Deposit Payment Responsibility Agreement." "Autologous" at that moment, is Greek* to me, but given my apprehensive state, I dutifully sign without fully understanding what I'm putting my name to, confident it's not harmful to my health. Later, I read the first sentence of the Agreement: "An autologous deposit is a collection of one's own

---

*Apropos Greek: "prostate" derives from the Hellenic for "stand before." It was coined by the French Surgeon, Ambrose Pare, a pioneer in prostate studies, to describe the gland's role as the "guardian of the bladder."

blood in preparation for a subsequent transfusion during surgery." I should have known that, but it's hard to get your mind to perform a language search when it has enough to do remembering its name.

Since there are a bunch of people waiting their turn, I settle in, hoping for a long wait, but am immediately directed into a cubicle to have my finger pricked.

This is the first time the nurse almost smiles. She congratulates me for having a high blood iron content as if I had personally dug up the ore, smelted it and mainlined the remaining metal. I explain that my doctor has put me on iron supplements.

"You'd be amazed at how quickly giving blood will deplete your iron," she lectures. "If it falls below a certain level, you can't give blood until it's back up again." Her joyful glare strengthens my resolve to never miss my daily iron intake. Besides, I wasn't going to give her the satisfaction of discovering my blood iron level was below par. Sorry, ma'am— you won't be gloating over my temporary anemia. As if I could do something about it.

"Mister Gottlieb?" The blood taker has come to get me. He leads me around the corner to the sterile abattoir. I follow as if in a trance.

I do not look at the other donees lest my legs leave me. (Needles, giving or getting, were part of the reason I dropped out of pre-med.) Instead, I stare at my technician's face hoping for some eye contact, hoping his incisors aren't extra sharp and a tad longer than normal, but he's focused on labeling tags and plastic bags.

"You've done this before?" I ask, a fun start for an instant bond. *If we're pals, you'll be extra careful, right?*

"Once or twice," he replies, concentrating on his tasks, a small smile starting under his moustache. Take your time, amigo. I've got all day. But my time runs out. He abrades my arm with a Betadine solution so vigorously, it feels as if he's removed a layer of skin. Good surgical procedure, but I'm hoping it doesn't augur the way he handles a needle.

I avert my eyes, examining the construction of the adjacent bed-couch as if I had to answer questions about how many springs it had, the servo-mechanisms it uses, the mill width of the chassis tubing. Every detail has to be memorized, because now I feel my upper arm being strapped, hear myself being told to make a fist, feel an uncomfortable tugging at my arm. I've stopped breathing.

"You can relax now, Mister Gottlieb."

I try to unglue my face, which has, to my surprise, formed a permanent cringe over my right eye, as if it were warding off a blow.

"Just keep pumping your fist every so often. It keeps the flow going."

Save the need for a skin transplant, the blood-letting isn't so bad. I even venture a quick peek at the tubing now red with my blood. I can do this four more times if only just to spite the Iron Lady.

I walk out into the day on a high from having survived, and having had a blood sugar fix from the blood bank's goody bar.

In fact, I'm so pleased the procedure was so relatively easy, I leave on the tacky, heart-shaped decal the technician sticks onto my shirt. So what if it's the heroic equivalent of a Good Conduct medal. I earned it. Also, if I suddenly become light-headed and pass out in the parking lot, the cute red heart will tell passersby what I collapsed from. Heroes can't be too cautious.

The next three pints of my blood were sucked out over a period of a month, in the same close-to painless fashion as the first time. The nurses and technicians were amiable enough, but distant. My lame jokes and nervous prattling never got past anyone's personal armor into friendly territory. Must be the line of work: if you've seen one vein you've seen 'em all.   The only possible fly in the bloodstream is that, at the second drawing, my blood iron content is markedly lower—still in the okay range—but enough for Iron Lady to predict doom by the time I get to pint five. *Thanks for sharing that with me, Madame.*

If I were bumped on the last go-around, it would give me but days before the operation to fortify my red blood cells, which would not be enough time. And not an option, either, because I didn't want to call down the operating date since that would leave me an added month of nibbling on my cuticles. Besides, my inner mission control was signaling a go, and I just wasn't sure I could get pumped up again if the operation schedule was aborted.

"You know," the Iron Maiden repeats herself as she revels in my lowered iron numbers, "It's just amazing how giving blood just sucks your blood dry like that! Why, I've had to send people away after their second pint. Took their blood a couple of weeks to get back into giving shape." She tries on a smile, but it's not her size. "Let's hope that doesn't happen to you."

I nod in agreement, quite sure she's hoping it does happen, sure she gets a frisson of delight when she has to put on a long face and tell someone their blood is below par. She can barely keep her ample bottom on her chair, so excited is she at even the hint of another rejection.

Before I suggest a change of occupation to her—which idea I reject since she might, out of spite, cook the numbers just to be able to bump me—I decide, instead, to increase my intake of meat, eggs, whole grain breads and cereals, green vegetables, nature's ironworks.

Old Iron Pants will never exult over my deficient hemoglobin, never enjoy that moment she no doubt lives for. I will not give her the satisfaction.

Pass the broccoli, honey.

Early May in Florida feels like late summer in the rest of the country, the better to try to heal my skin condition. Everything I'd read about psoriasis included ultra-violet light treatments as part of a therapeutic regime. Who needs a sunlamp in St. Pete! Every day, I'd lay face down on my balcony, letting the sun shine onto the back of my thighs. I'd read, talk on the phone, even work on a writing assignment on my stomach. But I had to lose an arm every few minutes to face an elbow up to the supposedly curative rays, which was an uncomfortable position to be in, a redundant reflection of my current condition.

I was beyond tears as these weeks went by and into a quiet sorrow I couldn't explain to anyone for it had no voice. No one can hear you sobbing inside. It can't be shared. It can barely be heard, and when you can hear it, it only makes you feel worse. Under the circumstances, a little depression would be normal, except that I was just about getting past the life-shattering effects of being down-sized in the workplace, and now my very existence was being threatened again.

It had taken me years to learn that I wasn't defined by my job, that it and I could exist apart thank you, that I had worth beyond my work. But the cloud that had finally lifted was now back, even more threatening than when I left the workplace to set out on my own. It shadowed my days in spite of all the sun that washed over me.

Physically, I'm walking my every-other-day three miles as if there were no pavement. The stricter than usual diet, and the more than recommended daily allowances of vitamins and minerals, all have conspired to make me look and feel as if I were in the best of health, lulling me into minimizing the severity of the upcoming operation. Feeling strong, it seems, inspires confidence which, in its turn, reinforces one's state of denial. And I'm in it, up to my neck.

You would think I would have reflected back on the rigors of a prior operation—the incredible discomforts, the breathtaking pains, the protracted healing process—used that experience to imagine what I'm in for at the end of May. But strength wins out. It muscles out any old medical nightmares; only empty-minded daydreams of rosy outcomes are allowed in.

I even begin to look forward to giving blood—to the exhilaration a touch of lightheadedness the procedure brings. I've never felt so full of life. Hell, I know men of my age who are old. I am not old yet, not at sixty, not feeling so damned good. I'm gonna be fine I tell myself, lying and praying at the same time.

Strength may lead to courage, but it can't chase away that tiny spider of dread that nests inside your head, the one who, hungry for attention, bites into your facade, its poison eating away at the fragile front you've erected, reminding you that this, indeed, could be the summer of your discontent.

Like the song says, "I'm laughin' on the outside . . . "

Five days after my fourth blood transfusion and eleven days before my radical prostatectomy brings us to May sixteenth and Doctor Mawn.

He sits on our side of his desk, close enough to touch. Once again, I have a bunch of questions, none of which I can recall. Rose is quiet, listening, on guard.

Tom jump starts the meeting. "Why don't I go over once again what you should expect . . . and if you have any questions after that I'll be glad to answer them."

Tom's informality tells me he trusts us as much as we do him. Either way, I don't think he'd resort to medical jargon if there were a lay term available. I'm sure he's aware that confronting prostate cancer is enough of a bruising and disorienting experience without adding more perplexities to an already chaotic situation.

I sit back and prepare to listen, but it's difficult to hear over the pounding in my ears, my heart beating as if I'd just run a couple of miles.

Tom begins. "The operation usually takes four-and-a-half hours, but it could go longer. No way to know until we're inside.

Plus there's some down-time after we remove the pelvic lymph nodes. They go to the pathology lab and we have to wait for the results."

"After the operation," Tom continues, "you'll be in recovery for a day or two, depends on how you're doing. You'll have a couple of drains coming out of your stomach, but they'll come out when it looks like the internal oozing has stopped. It's part of the drill. Absolutely normal."

"What about post-op pain?" I ask, suddenly reminded of the first few days after a hemorrhoidectomy done over twenty years ago, the seat of my troubles on fire and not enough drugs to extinguish the pain.

"My strongest recommendation is to go for the epidural anesthetic. I can't be any more emphatic." And I can't question his endorsement of this pain controller, since in my reading, I'd skipped the sections on anesthesia.

"That's what they give to women giving birth," Rose offers. "It's called a 'saddle block."

"You're right, Rose, and it works for men, as well. Really controls pain after the surgery. Also helps keep blood clots from forming in your legs." Tom looks at me for approval.

"You're the doctor," I remind him, affirming that I'm not about to micro-manage his operation. I don't want any of my helicopters crashing in the desert because I told him how to stage his assault. If I entrust you with the responsibility for my life, you automatically get the authority; it's a package deal.

"You'll be catheterized, too," Tom goes on. "For three weeks. It's awkward, but nothing you can't handle. It's a must, though. The *anastomosis*—surgeon lingo for a water-tight seal—needs time to heal. Oh, and make sure you've got enough diapers on hand. A lot of my patients buy them in quantity at the discount stores. They're expensive, and not covered by insurance."

He lets the overview sink in, then opens his palms to us for questions. I am still wrestling with the diaper concept. There is nothing left to ask at this point. I'm merely the passenger on this trip. Tom's got the wheel. I'll just sit back, stare sightless out of the window and worry my cuticles for the next eleven days.

The truth is, I didn't want to know anything more. I'd done my homework, answered all the questions, even forced myself to watch an actual radical prostatectomy on cable, performed by none other than the noted Doctor Walsh of Johns Hopkins, high priest of the prostate church. But even though I had learned that the first incision would run from that poor bastard's belly button to his pubis, an inch shy of the top of his penis, I had to hug my stomach with both hands as I watched, not letting go until the last staple was shot into place. Pretty soon I would be that poor bastard. Wake me when it's over.

"Will Bert need any in-home care when he gets back from the hospital?" Rose asks.

"Maybe one visit—depends on when he goes home. We can take care of that before he leaves the hospital. And from here on in, the hospital will handle all the paperwork, the pre-op scheduling, everything, right up to the big day."

Rose, though listening intently, looks to be off somewhere in caregiver's territory, contemplating the enormity of the whole affair, making plans, wincing.

"Everything's gonna be all right, Rose," Tom touches her shoulder. "I'm gonna do everything right." He looks into her eyes, his smile begging her attention, his Irish charm and reassurance working their magic.

Rose grasps his hand. "Promise me one thing, Tom." She waits till she has tacit agreement. "That the night before Bert's surgery, you'll only have one glass of wine with dinner. I want your hands to be steady tomorrow morning."

Tom solemnly promises, unable to stifle a grin.

Rose has injected a little bubbly into what could have been a maudlin set piece replete with tears. *Doctor, you will do everything to save my dear husband, won't you? Promise me you won't let him die! You won't screw up, will you!"*

We are all smiles as Tom hugs us both out of his office. His last words to me are, "You'll be glad you went with the epidural. See you in two weeks."

Daybook Entry: 5/16/94

<u>Patient: BG</u>

<u>Reason for Visit:</u> *Review procedure process, reiterate anaesthetic recommendation, post-operative expectations, and answer any last minute questions.*

<u>Prescribed:</u> *4 liters Golytely lavage day prior to procedure, plus Neomycin and Flagyl pre- and post cleansing.*

<u>Post Visit Thoughts & Observations:</u> *Conference was short, as were questions, and reassurances were mostly unnecessary. The Gottliebs, now that they're committed, don't seem to need much hand holding or awkward attempts at a positive spin. They have a realistic understanding of the disease, the survival process, even of the emotional rollercoaster ride they've been on, and will stay on long after the operation. All they want to hear now is that the operation was a success, that Bert was doing fine, and most important, that "it" was all out. I hope to God I'll be able to tell them that, not only after the procedure, but ten years down the road as well.*

My plate was full these days, but instead of having to juggle dates for shoots, editing, music, voiceover sessions, and interminable meetings, doctors and labs now had to be scheduled so they wouldn't conflict. I wondered, where would I, if still working, have found the time to go through this? Could I have worried about my job and my prostate (okay, my life) at the same time? Or is it ten pounds of crap I'd be trying to stuff into a five pound receptacle? How lucky not to have to engage in that conflict of interests. How lucky I had the freedom to waste days waiting for opinions, test results, information, relief. How lucky, indeed.

The calendar, though, did inform me that if I failed my blood iron test today, the eighteenth of May, I had just enough time to build it back up and deposit it before the operation nine days ahead. That would mean another trip to and from Tampa, another nerve-jangling finger prick, and a little less lining left in my esophagus—but no cancelling of the operation for want of a nail.

Even with this information, my stomach has more knots in it than a macrame rug as the Iron Maiden stares at the readout longer than usual, begging it to refute what she's seeing. Ruefully, she has to concede that I *just* made it. "You were *this* close," she says, the joy gone from her. "You were lucky this time, but that's the last blood *you'll* be giving for awhile!".

And now she is the gloatee and I can't resist. In my most saccharine voice and smile I tell her, "I'm sorry I ruined your day, Ma'am."

Our eyes meet. It's agreed: we hate each other. This is my fifth and last pint, my brass ring for the day, which puts me a couple of miles closer to P-Day, where I either die on the beach or make it all the way to the City of Lights.

The Surgicare Pre-Op morning resembles an Hieronymous Bosch tableau aptly titled *Medical Bedlam*. The noise, the crowds, kids crying everywhere, wriggling out of their parent's clutches to careen between and around the tightly-knit chairs and a dizzying assortment of legs, crutches and boom boxes, not to mention nurses and aides shouting over the din for their "Next!," present a nightmarish spectacle painted by a certified crazy.

Even my trusty crossword puzzles refuse to distract.

After a mercifully short wait, I'm beckoned into the swirl of nurses, aides and patients filling the equipment-laden hallway, and shown into one of the cubicles.

Each nurse carefully recites my name, rank and serial number, checking that I am whom I profess to be, not on any special medications, am not post-menopausal, and has me sign a bunch of releases, including, I suspect, the transfer of my first born to the hospital in the event my sickness insurance isn't sufficient.

My vitals are taken, I'm EKGd, then consigned to the hallway to wait for the anaesthesiologist, who shows up out of sorts and breath, sweat darkening his surgical greens. He looks to be a contemporary, and a New Yorker by the sound of him, all gruff exterior, inside a pussycat.

"Have you discussed the types of pain control with your doctor?"

"Yes. I'm going with the epidural," I answer without hesitation.

He nods agreement, smiles and makes a note in my file, which by now looks to be about two inches thick, enough to fill a book.

"Any questions?" He's already working on his next patient.

"Are *you* going to be my drug connection?"

"No."

"Too bad." I mean that as a compliment.

"Yeah, me too," he answers, which is about as close as a New Yorker gets to being warm and mushy. Then it's a sincere handshake, a wish for good luck and he's gone, and I'm done with the pre-op run-though.

I hurry down the hallway clutching the day-before-op instructions to my chest, a broken field runner adroitly avoiding unleashed children, scattered vitals' carts and scurrying hospital personnel, rushing toward the relative sanity of the real world.

The air outside, in spite of the oppressive morning heat, is sweet, untainted by the smell of urgency, anticipation and fear that pervade St. Joe's Surgicare section, and perhaps all such places, for all I know.

Sleep, that night, is fitful, interrupted by a recurring dream.

I'm running down a narrow, crowded street in an unfamiliar city and I trip over a vendor's metal stand, which, in painfully slow motion, begins its inevitable crash toward the ground, scattering strange implements everywhere. I'm embarrassed into wakefulness again and again, until my sweat makes the pillowcase feel as if it had been taken out of the drier too soon.

My inner analyst opines, I *sink your dream reflects emotions zat are being put through ze wringer, yah?*

No shit, Ziggy.

We've been invited to a lecture on prostate cancer at St. Joe's, which we probably won't go to, figuring that it's a little late for an overview of the subject, and that we probably know what's going to be said anyway. Either way, I've got prostate cancer overload. Adenocarcinoma has invaded every cranny of my existence. I've been eating it, drinking it, and when I could, sleeping with it. I wanted to hear no more about prostates except that mine was history.

I have my hair cut shorter than usual to look my best during the time I'm no doubt going to be looking my worst.

I somehow finish the character skeleton outlines and the first episode of a children's Saturday morning cartoon show—an effort doomed to failure since the basic idea is spectacularly out of touch, not to mention, trite. That's not to say I dragged my feet or gave the job second, or even third, shrift, but a mediocre concept can only be fleshed out and polished, at best, to a dull finish.

The work did, though, divert attention from my condition onto a cast of wacky characters involved in lots of *Pow! Bam! Boom!* It even buoyed me up enough to attend a script meeting the next day, where I bombed, not because the script wasn't good, but because I had had the temerity to change some of the characters' names—for the better, I thought, especially for healing some of the wounds the original names inflicted on the idea. Turns out, Mr. I-Put-Up-The-Money came up with the names. The fact that they didn't work, didn't match the characters, hindered the story line from ever making sense, weren't in the least clever, memorable or, worse yet, pronounceable, didn't matter; the big guy liked them. And as he raged on about our being philosophically incompatible and probably shouldn't be working together, my prostate functioned like a 10 milligram Valium. *You can't get to me, fella. I've been got to by something bigger than you and your turkey of a concept. And how can we be philosophically at loggerheads, when your head is up your ass. Besides, I'm too laid back right now to debate it with you, so there!*

In the parking lot, the producer who had hired me as scriptwriter, thanks me for being so cool and not losing my head, that he'll make sure I get my check, that with my incredibly perceptive and valid changes disregarded, the project now has even less of a chance to succeed, and how really well I took the rude rebuff from that cretin. And I'm wondering how I could write a script with so much violence (even though cartoons are mostly bloodless), while it's killing me to contemplate my own possibly bloody demise. After all, a major operation involves major risk. Any number of conditions could arise and cause you to be prematurely, if not permanently, fired from your profession.

My head might not have been buried in my bottom, but my heart was definitely in my mouth, leaving no room for such a mundane issue as a writing assignment..

The week preceding the operation is uneventful save for blowing off the prostate cancer lecture we'd been invited to. It was writ large on our calendar, but we conveniently ignored it. I know I did. Staring at the notation, I wondered whether I would have heard something I didn't already know. Truth was, I couldn't stand to hear anymore about prostate cancer at this time, this far down the road. I'd heard enough facts, chewed on the myriad questions a hundred times over, and had to accept the fact that answers wouldn't be available until well after the procedure. Besides, limbo was the perfect place to be on a lazy Sunday, where the New York Times Magazine crossword puzzle beckoned, a second cup of Tres Rios awaited savoring, and bathrobes were the uniform of the day. Save for a trip to the drugstore for diapers, bowel-cleansing solution, and pre-op antibiotics which are to be taken at the start, and after, the cleansing ritual, Rose and I don't venture out all week discovering, to our amazement, enough freezer-buried foods to live on for a month.

Being together, in virtual lockstep until I get rolled into the operating room, was all we needed. To call it togetherness doesn't begin to do it justice. If it were possible, we would have occupied the same space, because we knew that after the operation, we might never be together in the same way again.

The day before the day before, I dutifully prepare the six-and-a-half quarts of cleansing solution and refrigerate it because the instructions say it tastes better cold. Sure. Twenty-four hours before the big day, it feels as if this prostate business started just yesterday, not two months ago. Where does the time go when you're not having fun?

It is a clear day, though, this day before, and on a clear day, as the song proclaims, you can see forever.

Of course, on a clear liquid day, which this one is, from noon till six you can barely see beyond your knees, the lavage liquid having married you to the john. It's called Golytely, this internal cleanser—a smarmy name that left as bad a taste in my mouth as did the product itself. But according to Doctor Tom, it did the best job of scrubbing the gut clean, a must before the surgical procedure. So down the hatch, ridiculous spelling and all.

By the end of the day I am worn out from all the trips to the bathroom. Now that everything was all out, I was all in.

I crawl into bed and take Rose's hand. She squeezes mine goodnight. It is too late for anything but more fitful sleep, too late to turn back.

In my dream, I am dressed in surgical greens, standing over a draped figure, scalpel poised for the first incision. I make the cut and am surprised no blood is seeping out. Every layer of tissue, down to the capillaries, is textbook clear. I reach past the intestines, probing for something. When my fingers detect it, I wrench it out, holding it aloft over the patient, exulting in its glow. I have retrieved the golden walnut! Everyone in the OR claps. I join in the celebration after having pocketed the prize. A voice, the patient's, starts shouting, "Gimme back my prostate! There's nothing wrong with it! C'mon, put it back!"

I marvel at how he can talk with a breathing tube filling his throat. I search my pocket for the item, but when I turn to his midsection to put it back, I am shocked to see his stomach is uncut, intact.

"I'm sorry," I whisper to him. "It's too late."

He starts to cry, and I find myself crying, too, because I am him and flat on my back now, staring up into a posse of doctors hovering over me.

"What makes you think *your* walnut will be gold?" one of the doctors asks, then laughs, and then they all begin to laugh, and the laughter lingers in my consciousness even as I get out of bed, soaked and scared.

Whaddya think, Ziggy? Am I gonna be in stitches today?

Queasy is the operative word this morning. My stomach is jittery. Waves of nausea pound in my throat. My hands, normally rock steady, are shaking, keeping time with the quivering music in my gut. Even the cats sense that this day is different than all others. They mill around my feet rubbing their faces against my ankles, marking me with affection. When I reach down to stroke them and tell them I'll be back soon, I hear my voice cracking, feel tears welling up. They stare into my face, their innocent eyes begging for a reassurance I can't give myself, let alone them. But a can of Friskies diverts their attention long enough to allow me to shave without fear of stepping on someone's tail. I concentrate on trying to trim my sideburns squarely, but as hard as I try to make believe this is a day like any other, I'm not even close to successful. I feel like retching, but there's nothing to throw up. And my left eye is twitching—another rhythm added to this one-man band of emotional tics. Oh, what a beautiful morning.

"You packed everything?" Rose asks as we're driving into Tampa.

"Except for my tux."

"Your crossword puzzles?"

"Doesn't everybody when they're going to have a radical?"

"Your toothbrush?"

"And my floss, my super floss, my Butler Proxabrush, and a partridge in a pear tree."

"Funny man."

"I try."

For a long while, we're lost in our own bleak thoughts. Then Rose asks, "You okay?"

"Why? don't I look okay?"

"Yeah—except you're doing the speed limit."

"We've got plenty of time. Anyway, when was the last time anyone about to be executed *ran* the last mile?"

Another long silence.

"You'll call everyone after the . . . afterwards . . . Lori, your sister . . . "

"And all the pipers piping."

"Funny girl."

"I try."

"I love you, you know."

"Me, too."

Rose is inches away from tears.

"Hey! I'm gonna be okay."

"I know," she says, her eyes filling up.

I reach over and squeeze her hand. She squeezes back with a strength I didn't know she had.

"I'm gonna be okay. Really."

"You better be," she sniffles.

"Hope so." Now I've got the glooms, reality biting hard on my shell.

"You're gonna be okay," she lies, hopes, prays, consoles.

"I'm gonna be okay," I echo, without believing it. I turn on the radio and Imus is on, which wrenches a smile out of us. Then it's quiet, save for the macho banter coming from the speakers, until we arrive at St. Joe's. There are no words.

After registering, getting my ID bracelet, and forking over a large check to cover our end of the medical insurance, we're directed to a waiting room that's as cold as a tomb. I'm hoping it's not a portent.

Another couple shares the refrigerated space. We smile at them, and they at us, and that's it for communication. Strangers on a train to who knows where.

I lean over and whisper to Rose, "I wonder which of them is being chopped up this morning?" Anything to distract. But Rose won't play. So I try to work on a puzzle, but my brain is on vacation, refusing to come back and solve even the simplest clues.

A nurse comes to take the other couple away.

"Good luck," the wife says to us.

"You, too," Rose replies.

When they're out of earshot, I say, "I think *she's* the one. Major liposuction."

Rose slaps my hand—a chastising cuff.

"Actually," I continue, sensing she *will* play, "I've changed my mind. He's the one. Plastic surgery. Major jowl job."

Another slap. I grab her hand, kiss it and don't let go. I'm wishing we could sit like this forever, or at least until they find a cure for prostate cancer, but after what seems like too short a time, a nurse comes up and asks us to follow her. We're taken into a large ready-room and ushered into a small cubicle. I'm told to undress completely and don the requisite backward-tying gown and a pair of booties. By the time Rose has stowed my clothes and toilet gear and taken possession of my watch and wallet and asked me if I remembered to bring a pen for my crosswords (for the third time), the "shaver", a nurse's aide arrives. Rose is asked to leave—a strange request, since she has seen me naked before, like minutes ago—unless Madame Barber isn't too swift with a razor and doesn't want the caregiver fainting if I get nicked.

Turns out, I'm shaved to just above the pubic area, no further. My groin is even considerately covered with a towel.

Here, I thought I was in for some deep embarrassment as my privates are tenderly handled while a Personna Disposable explores their every curve, and all I get is a trim. The full job is no doubt a later procedure, done when I'm less susceptible to all the fondling that will surely transpire.

My relief, unfortunately, doesn't extend to this aide's obvious discomfort. Her strokes are tentative. They lack the feel of someone confident in their skills and comfortable in their work. And she can't look me in the eye.

Rose could have stayed.

After the nursing aide is gone, Rose comes back in, and is allowed to stay while a nurse hooks up my IV connection.

During the short procedure, I stare at Rose while she stares at the gruesome procedure. Yet she's not allowed to look at my stomach being shaved. Hospitals!

From the ready-room, I'm rolled into a hallway cum holding space where other patients on gurneys wait their turn for some sort of surgery. Rose hovers nearby.

A Doctor Richards comes up and introduces himself as the attending anaesthesist. His manner is pleasant, efficient and, as he reverifies my choice of painkiller, oddly calming. His quiet confidence washes over me, leaving me relaxed for the moment, sure I'm in good hands.

Doctor Tom stops by, and after patting me on the shoulder, holds his rock- steady hands out to Rose.

"I didn't even have *one* glass of wine last night." he reports, endearing himself to her by remembering their two week-ago conversation.

"When do you think you'll be . . . it'll be done?" Rose asks.

"Not for another four-five hours at least," Tom answers. Then he gently plies her hand from the gurney bar it's clamped onto, and takes it in his. "I want you to go home now. There's nothing you can do here. I'll call you when it's over. You'll have plenty of time to get back here to see him. Okay?" He forces a momentary smile out of her.

I can't begin to imagine what Rose will go through till she sees me again. Fact is, I can't imagine anything, because I'm on adrenalin overload and my brains are on temporary hold, merely recording events, feeling strangely dislocated. I'm here and yet I'm someplace else, possibly a safe house somewhere deep inside, walled off from worry, doubt, even fear.

Tom squeezes my shoulder. "I'll see you inside, Bert."

Rose kisses me and quickly turns away, her eyes brimming with tears. "I'll see you later!" I cheerily shout at her back. She nods as she starts to walk away, unable to say anything, but stops and turns and blows me a kiss. I do the same. My heart breaks for her, and for me. I already miss her, as someone begins wheeling me away.

While I'm being rolled through hallways and bumped into doors, banks of ceiling lights fill my point of view as if I were on a camera dolly shooting up, giving rise to the ridiculous notion that I've seen this television series before, only this time it's called "Tampa Hope."

In the OR a short, wide, black nurse is dressing down a young nurse. Something to do with having enough supplies on hand, a you'd-better-stay-on-your-toes-if-you're-gonna-work-in-*my*-OR tirade. The lady is obviously a hard taskmaster, a master sergeant who will breech no bullshit in *her* OR. I love hearing her. She fills me with confidence which, as common wisdom acknowledges, is half the battle. And I'm confident, with that hardnosed lady on the case, nothing is going to go wrong in *my* OR, either. As that thought takes hold, a river of calm washes over me. This is it—the moment all these months of anguish have led me to. Too late for tears or fears. Just let it be over.

Doctor Richards leans over me and reintroduces himself.

"I'm going to give you something to relax you," he says.

I remember nodding okay to him as he reached for something out of my sightline.

* * *

Chapter 5

Initiation Rites

While I did my best Rip Van Winkle imitation, expert hands invaded my innards in an attempt to win back my life. Best sleep I'd had in months.

Date: 5/27/94

Patient: BG

Postoperative Thoughts & Observations _(and, as it's been a long day, forgivable musings): Bert's operation was the only one I had planned to do today. There are a lot of routine operative procedures performed by urologic surgeons; a radical retropubic prostatectomy is not one of them._

The procedure was scheduled to start at 0730 hours, but I was awake at 0430 hours. I wanted enough time to take one last look at a video of a "radical" prepared by Doctor Thomas Stamey of Stanford University which stressed techniques somewhat varied from those of Doctor Patrick Walsh in his excellent Johns Hopkins' teaching video.

After oatmeal, toast and juice, prepared by my almost-awake wife, Tina, I was out the door before sunup.

It was still dark when I pulled into St. Joe's parking lot, and for some reason, it brought me back to how I felt when the "new" St. Joseph's had just opened its doors and I was still in training as a second-year urology resident at Tampa General Hospital. It would be two years before I'd be eligible to apply for surgical privileges at St. Josephs's, and I couldn't wait. Twenty-seven years later—the last 15 of which I'd been Chief of Urology *at St. Joe's—it still felt the way it did in 1967, full of promise and great expectations.*

The elevator to the sixth floor, where most of the urology patients were admitted, couldn't get there fast enough.

Surgeons are accustomed to making early morning rounds. They know that once the procedure is underway, they'll be confined to the operating room for most of the day, so it is of key importance that patients be seen and orders written before operations start.

Rounds finished, I met Bert and Rose on the OR floor for a last minute chat and to issue a few reassuring words. They were both alert and eager to get things rolling, but their eyes mirrored their anxiety. I would have worried had they not been apprehensive, considering the immensity of what would transpire today.

A final review of Bert's lab work, a check on last minute details, and it was time to look into the operating room.

The operating team was already assembled. It was a good team, utterly professional and rewarding to work with.

My Head Scrub was to be Missus Betty Carter, which assured a buttoned up OR, with everything and everyone running like the proverbial well-oiled machine. In Betty's OR, nurses had two choices: her way, or no way—the reason a few of the OR nurses preferred not to work with her, and why senior surgeons so often requested her.

Doctor Dan Richards, the anaesthesiologist this morning was busy setting up his feed lines and the epidural arrangement. Having done over fifty surgical procedures together, I knew Dan as a first-rate practitioner who works well under pressure. I also knew him as a friend. We often fish and dive together off Dan's boat, most fittingly named "Never Better."

The final member of our team is Doctor Leffie Carlton,

III—a most capable urologist in his own right, whose father, Doctor Carlton senior, pioneered thoracic and vascular surgery techniques at Tampa General and, as it happens, taught me basic surgical technique while I was in general surgical residency at that hospital. I was glad Leffie was assisting me.

The first part of the operation process is the laparoscopic pelvic lymphadenectomy, a procedure which doesn't involve the prostate.

The laparoscope allows us to remove and microscopically examine the pelvic lymph nodes for possible cancer spread, since they are the first place adenocarcinoma visits when intent on traveling. Thus, it is critical that the nodal status be known before surgery begins, or in a worst case scenario, doesn't.

The trick (a non-surgical term) is to painstakingly pick the nodes—soft, peanut-sized structures—off large arteries and veins, without nicking them.

The procedure is performed through a 10 millimeter incision (not quite half an inch) into which a long, relatively thin, tube-shaped camera is placed, deep into the peritoneal cavity. It illuminates the surgical site, and provides a vivid picture to the surgical team, who are viewing it on the monitor.

Once the nodes are plucked off the blood vessels, long, thin (5mm) dissecting forceps are then put in place. What makes this step dicey, and why infinite care is demanded, is that the nodes surround the obturator nerve, which, if cut, will result in a permanent weakness of the leg.

Today's nodal dissection went well, with no blood vessel or nerve problems. More important, there was "no evidence of metastasis," to quote our most able pathologist, Doctor Manuel Carta, who called us in the OR as soon as he had examined the frozen section and made his determination. This good news *brought on smiles that could be seen even under our surgical masks.*

Now we could begin, and at the same time, conclude, a process begun months ago. A skin incision was made in the lower abdomen from the pubic bone to the umbilicus. After entering the abdominal cavity, the wound edges were protected, retracted, and the prostate surface carefully exposed.

At this point in a radical, the oft-quoted urology adage always springs to mind: "If God wanted man to take out the prostate, he would not have put some of the biggest veins on top of it, and then stuck the whole thing under the biggest bone in the body."

To begin to free up the prostate, our next step was to cut the dense puboprostatic ligaments. These tough bands abut the deep dorsal vein complex, and despite every surgical precaution, we encountered some bleeding, which had to be brought under control before the operation could continue.

Although bleeding was venous (low pressure) rather than arterial (high pressure), it could nevertheless result in significant blood loss. Worse yet, venous bleeding is often more difficult to control because venous walls are thin and delicate, and thus difficult to suture. Though we were quick to control the bleeding, I was disturbed by Bert's having lost more blood than necessary. Doctor Richards, anticipating my concern, quietly assured me he was able to keep up with the replacement blood, and that we could continue without problem.

The next part of the procedure is of critical importance, as well: cutting the urethra from the apex of the prostate. Exceptional care must be taken to maintain as much urethral length (for continence) without injuring the nearby neurovascular complex.

Sparing the delicate nerve structures which control erec-

tile function is of equal importance, a fact first brought to the attention of urologists in 1982 by Doctor Patrick Walsh and his associates from Johns Hopkins. Their nerve-sparing technique was revolutionary, and remains the gold standard of surgical approaches, save when there's visible evidence of tumor invasion and removal of the tumor has to take precedence over sexual performance. Job number one is ridding the patient of his cancer. There's no toss-up about which road has to be taken. I'd rather have to tell a patient that he's lost his erection (a reparable condition in most cases) but gained his life in the bargain, rather than have to deliver grimmer news.

Once the urethra is free of the prostate, it and its capsule must be carefully separated from where they touch the rectum. This maneuver is, in most cases, a fairly straightforward one, because the dissection follows a natural cleavage plane known as Denonvillier's fascia.

Occasionally, though, the prostate and rectum manifest dense adhesions and scarring, largely obliterating the plane while raising the odds of a rectal injury. Because of that eventuality, I had Bert (as I do all my patients undergoing a radical) endure a Golytely bowel cleansing. If a rectal injury occurs while working on a fully-prepared bowel, it can be easily fixed. Conversely, if the bowel is not thoroughly clean, it may be necessary to perform a temporary diverting colostomy, a procedure to be avoided at all costs.

Today, there was a clear cleavage plane, so we were able to free the prostate and the attached seminal vesicles from the rectal area without difficulty.

The prostate was then severed from the bladder, removed and sent to pathology for analysis.

Bringing everything back together is the last critical task. With the prostate out, we are left with a bladder aperture about three times wider than the urethra, to which it must be joined. To create a proper fit and a solid seal, the bladder opening must be tailored to the urethra's smaller dimensions.

Unfortunately, the uretal orifices are extremely close to the bladder neck. As such, they must be identified and kept away from any sutures placed to reshape the bladder neck.

A misplaced stitch at this juncture could close off a uretal orifice, resulting in an obstructed kidney. In order to keep an eye on these orifices, a harmless dye—Indigo Carmine—is sometimes injected into the patient; it helps considerably in identifying the openings. It also turns the patient's urine a bright blue until it's excreted.

The bladder neck, having been tapered and tailored to size, is now ready to be sutured to the urethra. After the sutures have been stitched into a preset pattern, a Foley catheter is slid through the urethra and into the bladder. The sutures are then tightened, closing up the space once occupied by the prostate.

The catheter will be left in for about three weeks, to allow sufficient time for any incisions and sutures to have knit, avoiding any separation, which, if it should occur, could result in heavy urine leaking, scarring and a possible blocking of the bladder outlet.

Final steps involve putting the drains in place (which will collect blood, lymph or other fluids that can gather in the prostatic space), and closing the incision, which is done only after we are confident that all the packs, needles and instruments are out. To that end, nurses must count every single item that was (or could have been) used during the operation, and that count must be identical to the count taken before the operation proceeded.

While putting on the dressings and carefully securing the catheter, Leffie and I had to admit, although physically drained (the operation having run much longer than planned), we were *elated that it had gone well and that Bert's prognosis for a cure was excellent; the surgeon's ultimate reward.*

It was time to talk to Rose.

With some surgical outcomes, the hardest part of the procedure is talking to the family. Not today.

"Rose, there was no cancer evident in Bert's pelvic lymph nodes. His tumor appeared to be confined to the operative specimen. And our patient came through the operation very well indeed. I'm going to have an extra glass of wine tonight to celebrate. So should you."

Rose's grin and tears of delight were icing on the surgeon's cake.

* * *

Chapter 6

Post Hazing

I'm on my back, rolling and bumping along. My eyes flutter open with every lurch. I can't keep them open. My son's voice reaches me: "There's Dad!" I try to give a thumbs up in acknowledgement, but it is so difficult to think about which of my fingers is my thumb, I wind up giving him the finger, instead, to which he quietly shouts, "He's okay! Did you see it?" I think I hear Rose's voice indignantly, happily, tearily answer, "Of course, I saw it!" I think I'm back, but I think I'll just go back to sleep for awhile.

Four hands are busy adjusting things over my head, tugging on my bedclothes, rousing me back to life. Two faces, smiling, insistent, force me to cough. I have no legs, my arms are useless, and my head wants to flop over like a rag doll; the puppeteer is still on drugs. Coming out of general anaesthesia is a chore; you've got to struggle for every inch of consciousness. Time for another try at napping.

Hospital Progress Notes 5/27/94 T. Mawn
Vitals stable Blood chemistry presents high chloride levels (result of saline infusions) otherwise within normal parameters

"Bert! You have guests!" I'm being shaken into a dim consciousness. Rose swims into view with wet eyes and a dry kiss, replaced by son David and his wife, Asa, their mouths happy, their eyes wide at the sight of me. I cannot imagine what I look like, what the whole scene must look like. But I am alive and feeling no pain, in spite of being continually asked, "On a scale of one to ten, where would you put your pain at?" To which I always answer, "Does zero count as a number?"

I am also thirsty beyond measure. I've never been so thirsty—not after my first 5k race, not after a forced twenty mile hike across the lovely back forty of Fort Jackson, South Carolina, not even after watching *Tobruk*. I could drink the water cooler dry. I get a chip of ice. It is ambrosia. I, much like W.C. Fields, who never drank water if he could help it, have never tasted anything so delicious. I beg for more, doing my best imitation of Oliver Twist. I'm informed that until my stomach decides to join in the reawakening, too much liquid is a no-no. But I get another chip for a good performance, also, the whole cup of ice chips, if I promise to be good. Curiously, I don't cheat.

"Let's get you up now." Gail, one of the intensive care nurses is trying to extricate me and my accoutrements—the IV, the epidural, the catheter, a bewildering array of tubes—and prop me in a chair.

Rose hovers around me, grinning, smoothing my bedclothes. David and his and my friend, Mike—who has replaced Asa, who is out in the hall, recovering from the shock of seeing this kind of thing for the first time—chat with me about nothing important, and just as I am beginning to celebrate how good it is to be alive again, free of the awesome grip of anaesthesia, I begin to feel pain. Fire has started to lick at my insides, threatening to become a four alarmer. I beckon to my ever-vigilant nurse, "My pain's at 'five' and climbing fast!" She dashes to the phone, and before the pain moves up another number, Doctor Richards is there. With a reassuring touch on my arm and a hurried adjustment of the equipment, I'm almost immediately back to zero discomfort. Tom was right; the epidural is the Cadillac of pain killers.

I don't want Rose or my kids to go. I want this delicious visit to never end.

I also want to sleep. Everybody tiptoes out. See you tomorrow. My first night after the operation. I'm still here. Should be a good night.

I manage to sleep half the night, not in stretches, but at intervals of ten or so seconds. That's how long my "leg irons"—the automatically-inflating, elastic sock, leg massagers which aid circulation and prevent clots from forming while the patient is confined to bed—pause before recyling. When the pulsations begin, coiling upwards, squeezing you from ankle to thigh like two pet boas in estrus it isn't an unpleasant sensation; it's not soporific, either.

Come morning, I was stressed from lack of sleep and knew it, further confirming that I was alive, and if not exactly kicking, ready for some next steps.

A bed bath, dry shampoo, shave, change of gown and change of venue from bed to chair, courtesy of the supremely efficient, incredibly good-tempered, intensive care nurses, and I'm a foot closer to feeling human again. I can see it in Rose's eyes as she tiptoes in.

"You look a lot better than you did yesterday,"

"I feel a lot better, too," I say in my best Groucho voice, making sure I fan my hand out near my cheek.

"Are you in any pain?"

"No."

"No?" The look.

"No!"

Another look. I look back.

"Not a little prick?"

"Not a teeny-weeny-eeny prick."

Before we can continue this deep medical discussion, Doctor Tom breezes in. He gets me back in bed, pushes my gown up and lifts the bandages from my stomach. I chance a peek. Wrong move. Holding the wound together, there are metal staples running from belly button to infinity as if I were the result of one of Doctor Frankenstein's experiments. On top of that, there are drains on either side of my abdomen exuding bloody detritus. It's one thing to see this procedure on a television screen, quite another to glimpse it not a foot from your nose. It's a good thing I'm lying down. Tom, though, is grinning, obviously pleased at what he sees.

"You're coming along just fine, right on schedule . . . everything's looking good . . . and I think we're gonna get you outta here and into a room this afternoon."

Two giant steps.

Hospital Progress Notes 5/28/94, T. Mawn
Abdomen is soft A few bowel sounds Vital signs stable Moderate output from drains Urine output adequate & clear Epidural is functioning well - no pain, no complaints

As promised, I'm moved out of intensive care into a cramped room on the Cardiac Floor, this, with due apologies for there not being a bed available on the "right" floor, wherever that is.

Were it not for my roommate and his extended family, it wouldn't have been too bad dealing with day two—an endless procession of vitals taken, urine bags emptied, IVs replaced, and the ever-present pulsating stockings expanding and contracting, disturbing any efforts to sleep.

Unfortunately, said roommate was having problems with his pacemaker, a replacement implant, and doctor after doctor would try to explain why the problem was occurring, all with little success. Since only a thin curtain separated my side of the room from the other, I could hear every word, and not having the distraction of seeing the speakers, could focus on the sound of the voices. I heard fear and frustration when the patient spoke; his wife's voice begged to understand, prayed she didn't; the doctor sounded sad, in spite of his dry, clinical recitation of the facts, words that didn't even include "perhaps" or "maybe", let alone "hope." All the while, grown children, uncles, aunts, and assorted nieces echoed the doctor's dour forecast, a Greek chorus predicting doom.

It was a depressing distraction, but at least it kept me from wondering about my condition. Actually, there wasn't enough energy in me yet, nor enough gray cells on line, to contemplate my own outcome.

Doctor Richards broke the dreary spell by coming in to remove the epidural gear, supplanting gloom with fright. *Would the removal hurt? And afterwards, would I hurt?*

The spinal needle felt like a fine pin being slid out. I hadn't previously felt its presence, but my body seemed relieved that the foreign object was removed. My anxiety levels dropped several notches, and after a quick check of my nerve endings and finding no hint of pain, fell even further.

Doctor Richards then removed the intravenous connection stitched to the side of my neck, something (amazingly) I hadn't yet noticed. He explained that the connection served as a bypass into my jugular vein, through which the autologous blood could flow, far enough away from the crowded operation site to avoid any traffic jams. None of which made the ache in my neck any less irksome.

His equipment detached, Doctor Richards asked me if I recalled anything that happened in the OR while I was under anesthesia. When I told him I couldn't remember a thing, he seemed satisfied, shook my hand, wished me luck, and left.

It then came back to me: he had asked me the same question while he was adjusting the epidural flow in intensive care. I couldn't recall anything then, as I didn't now. But it left me wondering what *did* happen in the OR that I could possibly have recalled? Did I wake up mid-procedure and start singing? Did I thrash about, tearing at my IVs? Whatever could have happened for the doctor to have queried me about it twice? Another little something to roil the psyche.

Nightime in a hospital is torture. Doors are forever being

banged, bells are always ringing somewhere in the distance, lights are constantly being switched on and off, conversations float in incessantly. Alone with whatever morbid thoughts you can muster, your senses assailed every second of every drawn-out minute, you begin to think there's a plot afoot to keep you off-balance, a sensory-deprivation chamber they've consigned you to to keep your blood pressure up and your body awake—an insidious prompting to get you to want to leave the hospital as soon as possible.

Relief doesn't arrive until morning washes over the room, chasing the night away, delivering me to the third day, and a new room.

As I'm being settled into this bright, spacious room which, compared to the previous one, feels like a suite, I can't help but see my roommate struggling to stand up, gather his IV pole and catheter bag to go for a prescribed walk. He is in such discomfort he can't control his tears, but is obviously strong-willed, and will tough it out if that's what it takes to recover. Platitude or no, I feel his pain, every agonizing step of it.

John is a pipefitter by trade, a country songwriter by aspiration. A couple of days of beard hiding a face contorted with pain couldn't conceal his being a ruggedly handsome man. I'd have cast him as a good guy in a Western in a San Antonio minute.

He called himself a redneck, but underneath the country accent that related tales of outrageous fishing expeditions, beer-guzzling orgies and long-range hauls across the country in perilous semis, he was a special man, his sensitivies intact, his intelligence sizable. As he described his summer place, so evocative were his descriptions of the land, the sky, and their relationship to the house, he could have been Frank Lloyd Wright with a southern drawl.

Turns out the poor bastard had a radical, came through recovery with flying colors, was sent home to recoup and was doing so well, he was soon practicing his golf swing on the lawn. But minutes after his last swing, he was stricken with pain, and an accompanying high fever. It was enough to put him back in the hospital, where it was discovered that a hunk of his intestine had become clamped off, denying it an adequate blood supply, and what had been festering quietly, had become gangrenous. Result was they had to chop out a hunk of infected intestine, and thus his intense post-operative pain. His thirst couldn't be slaked until his bowels sounded like they were up and running. They couldn't palliate his pain, either, since he had been talked into patient-administered anesthetic. It's a nice sales pitch: anytime you want more painkiller, just push the button. What they fail to tell you is that if you use up your meager allotment of anodyne too soon, your pain will rage at full tilt until the goddamned machine will allow you another slight spritz of relief.

I counted my epidural blessings.

My first walk around the hospital corridors is not nearly as bad as I imagined it would be. Save for being slow, unsteady, seriously wetting the front of my gown (a common occurrence no one pays mind to, relieving me of some measure of embarrassment), and trying to manage the IV pole and its accoutrements, Rose and the accompanying nurse tell me I'm doing just fine in that tone of voice one uses to children and lunatics. Here I am, bent over, tacking from side to side like a marinated mariner, and they're telling me I'm doing fine. If this is fine, I dread to think what so-so looks like. At the same time, I realize that more of me has returned, reaffirming that I am indeed alive, amongst the walking wounded perhaps, but achingly and joyously alive. I had survived the battle. Only one question remained: Had I won the war? It nags at me even when I'm back in bed, even as I realize how utterly fatigued I am from my short walk.

People come and visit. Flowers fill every available space. Rose is ever there. Doctor Tom checks in. I'm doing just fine, especially since the robotic socks have been taken off now that I'm ambulatory.

I've got a hospital acquaintance, too. Tom Hall, a Tampa native, noted public relations person, and all-around nice guy, is on my floor, recovering from a heart valve replacement. The valve failed while he was in Manhattan, yet he flew back to St. Joe's to have it repaired. His trust in this area's physicians and facilities reaffirmed my choice in sticking near to what I realize I'm now calling home. Being able to bump into a new friend like Tom, as both of us struggle our awkward way along the corridors, seems to make my transplant to Florida more complete, with me more connected to the Tampa Bay community, far less an alien Yankee.

A second walk, and I'm standing straighter, walking rather than dragging, and I'm beginning to feel that I am indeed doing fine—a lot finer than my roommate, who has the mispleasure of a visit from his surgeon.

From what I can make out, he is being told he just has to wait it out, with no comfort from additional drugs, or from the doctor, who never quite entered his patient's space, and only spoke to the air or at his charts, never to the patient, not to his face. Two minutes of painful frustration, this non-visit.

I feel like shouting after him: *You insensitive bastard! Just because you can't give him medical relief, couldn't you have squeezed out a couple of ccs of understanding, spared a few uppers of encouragement? If you'd bothered to look, you'd see his pain isn't just in his bowels? Call yourself a doctor?!*

I am so angry, it takes me a moment to realize *my* doctor is standing at my side.

"How's it going, Bert?" Tom asks as he checks my charts and his handiwork.

"I'm fine, Tom, but the guy across the room—John—is in a bad way," and still in high dudgeon, blurt out what just transpired, adding my take on what the doctor should have dispensed.

Tom promises to talk to him before he leaves. When he does, I can't hear his words, so quietly is he talking, but I can see the effect on John. Maybe it's my imagination, but his face has become unscrewed, his body more at ease.

After Tom leaves, John shouts over to me, "Your doctor! He's a helluva doctor!"

"Tell me!" I shout back, thrilled that John, for the first time this day, sounds stronger and obviously heartened.

Day three, despite common wisdom predictions, isn't the worst day after all.

Hospital Progress Notes 5/29/94 T. Mawn
Temp 100.3 Abdomen soft Some bowel sounds Minimal
output from drains Hemocrit okay. Stable vitals Urine output
adequate & clear Minimal discomfort Path. pending

Night three is an eyewitness news experience.

I'm awakened around midnight by loud voices. Sounds like a party is being held in the corridor. What happened to rest for the recuperating?

I ring for the nurse. She comes in and closes the door behind her. "Just stay in your room, Mister Gottlieb," she whispers. "We're, uh, doing our best to sedate him."

"Sedate who? Why? And who are all those people outside?"

"Friends come to help. He's been shot . . . won't cooperate . . . high on something or other . . . guards should be here soon. Keep the door closed!" Nurse slips out.

Keep the door closed? To shut Mister Drug-Crazed Lunatic out? Or to prevent me from hobbling to the rescue, overpowering the huge madman (from the sound of him), with my IV pole and catheter bag?

The guards arrive. So do the police. I hear them trying to reason with the patient even though he's screaming obscenities at them. Scuffling sounds ensue. "Hold him!" A lamp breaks against a wall. A heavy metal object clangs loudly and repeatedly as it falls. A stampede of feet pounds the vinyl, running away towards the nursing station. The echoes of the fracas hang in the air. Film at eleven.

I buzz for a nurse.

"Yes?"

"What happened?"

"Are you in pain, Mister Gottlieb?"

"No, I'm giving birth!"

"I'll be right there!"

When the nurse bursts her way in, I allay her anxiety about my condition by informing her that all I want to know is what happened.

"Oh, you mean the guy who was shot who ran out of here?"

"Yeah, *that* guy."

"He tore out his IV . . . ripped off his gown and . . . " She starts to giggle. " . . . left the premises like the day he was born." We both giggle over this picture.

The best thing about this made-for-TV episode is that I haven't thought about my drains, staples, catheter, frailty, or any of the other discomforts and worries that seem to inform my life, so caught up have I been in the pulse-pounding human drama that had just unfolded outside my door. Distraction has its virtues.

John, amazingly, has slept though the entire flurry of excitement. The healing power of words; my doctor as shaman and priest. Yes.

Sometime before morning I am awakened by an overwhelming urge to urinate, an overpowering, burning effort to void, the force of the surge threatening its way past the catheter (the preferred route out), and I thoroughly wet myself.

After handing me a fresh gown, the obliging night nurse opines that I probably had a bladder spasm. A spasm? To my mind, a spasm was an uncontrolled shake of short duration, a last spastic jerk or two. The act my bladder performed resembled more an old washing machine run amok during its spin cycle, threatening to self-destruct, until it suddenly stops thrashing about with a last, loud quiver. But you can shut off a washing machine and walk away . When your bladder is running amok, out of your control, there's nowhere you can go, no off switch.

My first question to Tom would be whether this episode was a portent of some unforeseen medical calamity.

What a parade of events on this third day, which it turns out, is Memorial Day '94. Where's a marching band when you need one?

Early on the morning of day four, Doctor Tom arrives, grinning with good news. The pathology report shows no evidence of metastasis in either the seminal vesicles or the lymph nodes. It was, though, about twenty-percent larger than predicted and full of "hot spots"—clinical shorthand for about-to-run-wild cancer sites.

I thought: not exactly like the oversimplified illustration (courtesy of a pharmaceutical firm), of a walnut-sized prostate in its various degenerative stages that sits on the side of your desk.

What I said was: "Not exactly like the pictures, huh?"

"Not even close," Tom agrees. "Your prostate weighed in at eighty-five grams. Filled the palm of my hand. And there was one close surgical margin near the base on the right side. But I think we did all right. We'll be keeping on eye on it, though."

I didn't exhale at this news. Also, I wasn't sure of what "surgical margin" meant. As far as I knew, margin implied room—margin of error, the margins on a page—space to negotiate. But what I inferred from Tom, was that a margin, surgically, meant a little too close for comfort.

But he would watch it. And I would wait.

In spite of a successful radical, I'm backed into watchful waiting, forced to take a lot longer view than I had planned on, forced to accept the idea that with prostate cancer, nothing is cut and dried. You're not cancerful one day and cancerless the next. What you are is forever on alert, watching carefully, waiting for signs, hoping there aren't any, and if there aren't, you're pulling a punch in the air and beginning the vigil all over again.

The upside of day four is that it can only get better.

I tell Tom about my bladder incident. He allows as how muscle spasms will occur now and again until the bladder realizes it's been sidelined for awhile, the Foley catheter having been sent in as a substitute lineman.

"The bladder has incredibly strong muscles. When it spasms, it's strong enough to force the urine out between the walls of the catheter and the urethra, which is a helluva tight squeeze. So you can imagine the strength that bladder muscles can bring to bear. But it might not even happen again. I wouldn't worry about it unless it continues."

Me worry about bladder spasms? Not when there's a surgical margin to fret over.

I don't forget to ask Tom about Doctor Richard's questioning me twice about whether I recalled anything of the procedure. "He has to ask it," is his answer. "It's a standard part of the anaesthesiologist's drill. Nothing to worry about."

Chalk off one less concern.

Tom leaves as breakfast arrives, a disappointing array of plastic dishes and industrial-strength food.

The given is: hospital food is the same, whether it's at St. Joe's in Tampa or as I recall, at Valley Hospital in Ridgewood, New Jersey, and most probably everywhere else.

Is there a cabal of executive hospital chefs in the pockets of the major food companies and the local provisioners—an ultra-secret, Mayonnaise, White Bread and Jello Group that actually decides to serve up bland, overcooked, unappetizing food to a captive, helpless audience? Or is it lack of food management skills that orders up a plethora of comfort foods and ensures they're cooked without a soupcon of satisfaction?

My suggestion: figure out how an authentic Greek diner (especially one in New Jersey) is run. There must exist a universal, authentic Greek diner recipe book and menu planner, because no matter which diner's leatherette seat you slide into, if it's Sunday night (at least in New Jersey), you can count on enjoying Cream of Turkey soup—a viscous veloute thinned ever so slightly by a sturdy, aromatic turkey stock, enriched with a scattering of white rice, shreds of turkey meat, and a few slivers of sweet red pimento. Same delicious soup in Teaneck as in Saddle River. Same incredible variety of choices, all served 24 hours a day. *A bowl of Creamo, Christos! Two lamb shank dinners with the oven-roasted* potatoes! *And a western, home fries, and burn the toast! What'll ya' have, folks?* Heaven!

How do they do it? How do they turn out hundreds of satisfying breakfasts, lunches and dinners round the clock? And more important, profit enough to buy pricey homes, and be able to vacation in Greece in the bargain?

Perhaps hospitals should consider hiring authentic Greek diner management to run their kitchens. Ambulatory patients would be dancing in the aisles between the beds; those confined to their beds would at least have their taste buds leaping around enthusiastically. And the HMO's should eat it up since it could become another delicious profit center.

After breakfast, a complete toilet ritual, and a longer-than-ever-before walk, I'm physically drained, yet full of an inner energy, an awakening of yet another part of me. Feels like all the synapses have finally come on line. Except for the parts that are busy healing, the rest of me is itching to go on to the next step.

"Hey, handsome," Rose remarks when she sees me shorn and shining, hospital gown hidden under my casually-elegant seersucker robe.

I *am* doing fine! I can see it in Rose's eyes, her smile, and her kiss—now firmly planted on my lips, not pecked gingerly on my forehead as if I might break under the pressure..

"This is for you," Rose says and hands me a gift-wrapped, oversized, colorfully-painted mug filled with flowers, lollipops and best wishes from my dentist's office.

When I try to read the card, my eyes fill up, blurring the words, splattering the ink. These thoughtful people, strangers really, have so touched me with their caring gesture, I'm left bawling uncontrollably. Trying to explain my conflicted emotions to Rose only results in more tears. She holds me, strokes my head, encourages me to cry it out. As my sobbing abates and the tears slow to a trickle, underneath the warmth and love that even mere acquaintances can now fill me with, there's a certain hollowness, a lonely space that refuses to cede what I had to surrender to survive. It is a sad place best stayed clear of. I knew, if I ever ventured into its darkness, I'd have to fight for my life to get out, and I didn't have the strength or the inclination to go there, just yet, if ever. My days of battling dragons were over.

Well, Ziggy? Am I, indeed, doing fine? Or am I certifiable?

Hospital Progress Notes 5/30/94 T.Mawn
Temp to 101.2 POD #3 Chest clear No pain Leaks around Foley when up No major drainage Active bowel sounds No flatus yet.Path results: no evidence of metastasis in either lymph node - no evidence of malignancy in seminal vesicles and sur-

rounding tissue Prostate presented moderately differentiated ad-enocarcinoma Gleason 2+3=5 with bilateral involvement The right margin of resection at the base of the gland is involved by tumor

After five days, I'm not only doing fine, I've got the hospital routine down pat: learned to sleep between vitals visitations; accepted the noise and other intrusions as normal; given up embarrassment for a lifetime.

The day would have slipped by unceremoniously except for my drains coming out, not an unhappy event. As the nurse removes my bandages, in walks a doctor sans white coat, announcing that he is, indeed, a doctor—Bruce Crowell by name—and a formidable medicine man. By the sound of him he's a southerner; by the look of him, a throwback to another time: suit circa 1952; tie from the planet Garish; hair a cross between Don King and Kramer. I love him.

He is raucous, giddily alive, and so swift and sure, the drains are out before I can say ouch. All I have time for is a sudden, noisy, involuntary exhalation of breath. To which the good doctor responds, a Cheshire cat grin lighting up his face, "Don't you say that about my mother!" At which point he flies out the room, leaving behind a smile that lasts the rest of the day, and me wondering who that unmasked man really was. It even makes the meat loaf tolerable.

Hospital Progress Notes 5/31/94 T. Mawn
Temp 99.4 Urine clear Passing flatus Minimum discomfort Abdomen soft (Jackson Pratt drains removed) Bun 2 CR 1.0 Relayed path results to patient

"Your staples are coming out today," Doctor Tom announces the morning of my sixth, and as it turns out, last day in the hospital.

In spite of the fact that I know their removal has to be simple and painfree, and that it's a positive step in the recuperative process, I can't help but envision a giant staple remover pinching and tugging at my tender flesh in an effort to spread and loosen the construction-sized staples.

If I had had the good sense not to concentrate on each staple (I didn't dare peek), I probably wouldn't have felt even the few slight stings that accompanied their extraction.

While new dressings are about to be applied, I screw up my courage enough to sneak a look. To my surprise, the edges of the wound, though understandably swollen, are firmly sealed, and neatly bordered by a score of red-dotted holes marking where the staples had been; a grotesque closeup from a horror film, repellent and fascinating at the same time.

Dressings done, Tom looks up and tells me, "I'm sending you home today. You're well enough to leave. And you'll do even better at home."

The idea of home is both wonderful and unsettling; there's no place like it, but at home, you have to watch yourself. At the hospital you're watched by an entire staff. *What if something dire occurred at home? Like what? Like who knows? Some complication! Hell, it's half an hour into Tampa! You know what can happen in that time?! Why didn't you get a doctor closer to home?! Because you wanted the best! Yeah, but you can't expect your doctor to drop everything and come rushing over in an emergency! You've gotta get there! Hit a couple of bridges and you're looking at maybe three-quarters of an hour! A lot could happen in fifteen minutes for chrissakes!*

"I'm also recommending a home care nurse visit you tomorrow," Tom adds. "She'll check you out, make sure you're fully-oriented, the whole nine yards."

"You're the doctor," I quip, seeing he is emphatic about this, wondering if I've missed anything while I was visiting Schizoidville.

"In two weeks, since I'll be away, your catheter will be removed by Doctor Carlton, who assisted in your operation. Any problems, questions, anytime, call him. My office'll set up the appointment."

"In the interim," Tom continues, "don't lift anything heavier than your urine bag. No straining, either. Stay on your stool softener. Otherwise, normal diet, plenty of liquids. Shower whenever you want. I'm writing you a prescription for pain. And take your antibiotics religiously."

I nod, hoping some part of my mind is retaining all of these instructions.

"Any questions?" Tom asks before leaving.

"What about the rash on my back?" I hadn't seen it (or for that matter, even felt it), but Rose had, and told me to ask about it.

"It's probably your skin's reaction to the sheets you've been lying on. I think it's the soap the hospital laundry uses. Some people are sensitive to it. It'll clear up soon. Nothing to worry about. Have the nurses shown you how to use the leg bag?"

Yes, I nod, remembering how casually they talked about it, how detached their words. I wanted someone to say: "Gee, what a terrible thing, having to pee in a bag strapped to your thigh." I didn't want facts; I wanted pity, commiseration, someone to acknowledge the awfulness of it.

My chagrin must have been obvious, because Tom squeezed my arm and put his face close to mine. "Bert. This is temporary. Two weeks and you'll be rid of it. Okay?" Another squeeze.

Must be doctor-patient transference-magic because the blues have flown away.

I offer Tom my hand. "Tom. Two things: Have a great vacation, and . . . thanks."

Tom shakes back. "You're gonna be fine, Bert."

In spite of my doubts, my fears, my pains and all my other

my-my's, I believe him.

Hospital Progress Notes 6/1/94 T. Mawn
Slight temp after drains were removed Skin staples removed
Incision is clean Home today Rx:Trimethoprim 100 mg. Bid
Darvocet N100 prn for pain

Leg bag rigged, dressed in mufti for the first time in five days, I'm an impatient patient waiting for the wheelchair to come and wisk me away. The only thing left to do is say goodbye to my roommate. We are war-time buddies, he and I, bonded forever by our shared battle against a common enemy, and now recuperating from our wounds. And though we have nothing much in common save our humanity, we've touched each other in a way few men get the opportunity to.

We hold each others hands as we shake goodbye.

"John, you old dog. You know why you're gonna come outta this okay? (John's idiot doctor had told him to count on only a limited few years.) Because you're too ugly and too mean to die!"

"Yeah, heaven is too fulla rednecks already."

"Damn straight, pal." A long pause.

"You know, Bert, once in a while, even a shitkicker like me has the good fortune to meet a real mensch. I've sure been privileged to meet you and your wonderful family. Now get your ass home, you Yankee carpetbagger. And don't let me hear about you gettin' sick again."

I have a hard time holding back my tears as John and I awkwardly hug each other for the first and last time.

Mensch! From a redneck yet. There is hope.

Rose is driving as if "Glass: Handle With Care" were stenciled across my forehead, even though I am in no danger atop my whoopee cushion, which is doing a fine, if squishy job of absorbing any bumps that slip past the car's shocks. But the world—not to be confused with highway traffic, of which we're the slowest—seems to be moving too fast. What I thought a reasonably quick gait in the hospital, more aptly resembles a snail's pace outside it. The few steps from wheelchair to car seemed to take forever. I wanted to erase that memory and get up to speed as quickly as possible, ."Rose! Can't you go a little faster? I'm not gonna break!"

Discharge Report: Dr. Mawn, 6/2/94
Patient: Bert Gottlieb (Admitted 5/27/94)
Brief History: This is a 61-year old male who was admitted following a positive biopsy of a prostatic nodule which measured approximately 1.5 cm. on digital rectal examination, PSA 7.5 Ng/ml. Biopsy returned as moderately-differentiated adenocarcinoma. Prostate was ultrasonically determined to be 70 grams. PSA density was 0.106. Bone scan and CT scan of the pelvis were negative for evidence of spread. Chest X-ray was normal. He is allergic to Penicillin. He donated autologous blood.
Hospital Course: Patient underwent laparoscopic pelvic lymphadenectomy and radical retropublic prostatectomy on the day of admission. At the time of surgery, considerable oozing was encountered, primarily from the dorsal venous complex. It was necessary to replace both autologous blood, and in addition, bank blood. Excised prostate was over 80 grams.
Postoperative: Patient tolerated his procedure well. He was observed first in ICU and then in progressive for two days. Anaesthesiologist controlled his pain with an epidural catheter. His sutures were removed, he ambulated well, and was able to tolerate a surgical soft diet prior to discharge. The Jackson-Pratt drains were removed the day prior to discharge, and skin staples

were removed the day of discharge. The catheter will be left in place for 2 weeks.

Instructions: *Patient has been instructed in both bedside and leg bag use. He will be seen by a home health care nurse to assist him in the postoperative course. At the time of discharge, BUN was 5, creatinine 0.9 and hemoglobin 12. He was advised to avoid heavy lifting or straining. May shower. Regular diet. He will take Metamucil for his bowels and, in addition, will have Darvocet-N 100 prn for pain. Patient has a rash, primarily involving his back, which didn't look to be drug related. However, Ciprofloxacin, which was used during the hospitalization, was discontinued. He will receive instead, Trimethoprim 100 mg. b.i.d. He is to be at Dr. Carlton's office in approximately two weeks to have the catheter removed, as I will be unavailable at that time. He will see me two weeks later.*

Pathology Report: *Returned as moderately-differentiated adenocarcinoma, Gleason score of 5. There was no evidence of lymph node metastasis. Perineural involvement was not identified and the vesicles were not invaded. There was one close surgical margin on the right side near the base. He will be followed carefully in that regard with continued PSA testing and focused visits, even though we are finding that close margins don't always have clinical significance, since patients who have a recurrence, don't necessarily have a close surgical margin. Follow-up pathology studies often reveal that of the inked margins, many are unreliable in at least 30% of the analyzed specimens. Thus, the prognosis is basically the same for patients who have close margins as for those who don't. This is not to say that physicians should discontinue their continued post-operative follow-ups. I will be seeing Bert twice a year through the 5 year window, then once a year for five more years. If there is no recurrence within this 10 year window, the odds against a recurrence happening will be low enough for me to say Bert is finally cured.*

Chapter 7

. . . But No Cigar

It is good being home, except the apartment seems larger. Or is it that I feel smaller? Our wall-to-wall mirrors—the ubiquitous Florida decoration—decide the question; the bathroom scale cinches it. I've lost fifteen pounds. I'm what I weighed in college. It's hard to imagine that five days without food, or six days if you include the Golitely day—all right, hospital food *is* food (a stretch), so make it three days—would result in all that weight loss. The missing prostate couldn't account for it. Even allowing for, say, five pounds from the forced fast, it still leaves ten pounds unaccounted for. Blood loss? What was lost was replaced, and then some. It's a question for another time, this case of the missing pounds, because now bed beckons. I'm worn out from the ride home and my head isn't quite on straight, because I have the absurd thought that perhaps the good doctor did a little liposuction while he was rummaging around inside me.

If home is wonderful to be in, bed is even more so: crisp sheets (a giant, absorbent pad lying discretely under them, just in case), three pillows, king-sized leg room.

Sleep is not so terrific. After lying down, I quickly realize I'm consigned to remain on my back lest I foul up the catheter tubing by turning on my side too strenuously. The truth is, I'm scared I'll screw it up and create an emergency plumbing crisis. Understand, I was born without mechanical genes; in kindergarten, I flunked Tinker Toys. But, like the adult I'd like to think I am, I tell myself it's temporary, only two weeks to go (a lousy choice of phrase), but that fails to satisfy the stunning need to get rid of this device.

When sleep does come, it is fitful; muscle spasms and short explosions of pain jolt me awake through the night. The body is no doubt reliving the trauma of the operation, twitching and recoiling at memories of its skin being pierced and sliced, its blood vessels severed. The invasion into its delicate, intricate, born-to-remain virginal territory, where pain is not recalled consciously, is never forgotten by every cell that has been unfortunate enough to be caught in the onslaught.

I am no help to the sleeping process either, because, in between spasms, my inner clock keeps waking me to check the urine level on the catheter bag. Morning can't come too soon.

Breakfast in bed—bacon, eggs, buttered toast, coffee with cream—fussed over by my favorite short order cook, is obviously designed to put some weight back on me, damn the fat and cholesterol.

"Best breakfast I ever et, woman."

"You could use a little fattening up, mister," Rose says, starting to cry as she's looking at me.

I grab her hand and pull her toward me.

"Come here, you, and gimme a kiss."

After an awkward peck, thanks to our having to maneuver around the breakfast tray and catheter equipment, I whisper: "Hey, I'm alive. Everything's up from here."

I don't believe a word of what I'm saying, nor does Rose. We know there are too many potential pitalls to believe with any conviction that up was the direction we were headed in. The awful truth of this has us both crying.

"You look like shit, my dear," Rose manages to get out between sniffles.

"Of course I do, my darling. It's been a week since I've

really cleaned up. Give me an hour and I'll return your handsome prince to you. But first, kiss the frog again."

Before I get into the shower stall, the catheter line has to be disconnected. I do it, naturally, outside the shower and wind up dribbling urine all over the bath mat. A liquid learning experience.

The warm water feels delicious on my body, except for where it splashes on my groin. There, everything is too sensitive to bear even a gentle rain. Instinctively, I protect my parts with my hands, and for the first time, chance a good look down south.

I am not ready for what I see. My testicles and penis are black and blue, no doubt bruised from the operational procedures. The incision site meanders down from my navel in a squiggly line, which I assume will straighten itself out as the swellings come down and the tissue is healed. Yet for all my understanding, the sight of the family jewels, now so tarnished, is still appalling.

As I'm drying off, having reconnected myself to the catheter bag (which, now that it's my constant companion, I christen "Rover"), I catch a glimpse of my back in the mirror. It is a vicious red hive, spread completely from neck to butt; the rash they spoke about in the hospital. *But nobody said it was gonna be this big!* It dwarfs the crotch colors. I swear to myself that if my skin returns to anything nearing normal, I'll never eat a strawberry again .

Shaved, mustache trimmed, hair combed, teeth polished, cologne applied, I am as close to royalty, lack of a silk robe notwithstanding, as one can get, except it has taken two hours to get there, and the trip has left me fatigued.

As Rose helps me into bed, she allows as how I am, indeed, a princely sort of chap, but a bit of a dunce for wearing myself out primping.

"I won't fuss so much if you stop looking at me as if I were a corpse."

Now we're both crying again.

"Stop your sniveling, woman, and get to work," I snivel.

"You stay in bed, hear," Rose snivels back.

"I love you."

"Me, too. See you later."

I lie there, thankful that the war is over, rueful that the battle has just begun.

When the visiting nurse arrives, it is like the hospital come to call. She is all in white, down to her Reeboks, and unlike the cadre of nurses at St. Joe's, as stiff and unimpressionable as the starch in her uniform.

She takes my vitals, checks the wound site, and recites the litany of do's and don'ts as if I weren't in the same room. I am seemingly less important to her than all the charts and forms she dutifully has me sign, almost a non-person, not a soul who's been through merry hell.

What would it have cost to reassure me of my progress, perhaps stroking the insecurities she must realize exists in patients like me? Would a few words of solace, even if they were, at best, an exaggeration, have breeched the ethics of her profession? Like a call girl, she is efficient, bloodless and can't wait to tuck the money in her bra and get on to her next assignment.

Perhaps it's my fault. I tend to put up a great front, which might have led her to believe I had it all together, was so strong I didn't need any emotional hand-holding. Even so.

I would have declared the visit a waste of time, save for the fact that she showed me a most elegant way of emptying the urine bag, something I would never have figured out on my mechanically-challenged own. Everything else, up to and including how to apply the Betadine salve to the meatus to forestall infection, had been shown to me by the St. Joe nurses.

So dispassionate is she, that after the door closes behind her, it's as if no one has been to see me. I stand in the vestibule, weeping, wondering whether my teariness isn't just a concomitant of the post prostate blues, a condition which will ease up in time.I am wrong. It turns out that this is the beginning of my "weepy" period.

Like most men, I prided myself on being stalwart: didn't cry when Bambi's mom went to deer heaven; didn't shed a tear at John-John's dad's funeral cortege; was even dry-eyed at my son's wedding, a six handkerchief affair for his mother and sister.

The most sorrowful events failed to stir my tear ducts. I admit I blinked at times, my heart heavy when tragedy struck, but crying, never.

There were two exceptions. A lifetime ago, on leave in Paris, I lost it after hearing Renata Tebaldi sing *Un Bel Di*, prompting a French dowager to remark to her companion, "I thought Americans were heartless." And at my mother's passing, I couldn't mouth the prayer for the dead for the tears that flowed and wouldn't quit for hours afterward.

But now the sight and plight of utter strangers—Rwandan refugees, holocaust victims, any and all people who suffered—had me bawling. The slightest touching incident between family members, friends or mere acquaintances, and I'm gulping and dabbing at my eyes. These days, a gorgeous sunset is enough set me off. And there better be a full tissue box handy when Demi Moore is touched by Patrick Swayze's ghost. From the moment life cues the strings, I can feel the waters welling up and my heart begin to pump out tears.

I've taken to wearing sunglasses so no one can see my constantly-reddened eyes, never go out without pockets-ful of Kleenex. Yet even as my eyes blur and my nose begins to run, I rejoice in my new-found openness.

In the days before the catheter is to be removed, I work at regaining my strength by taking Rover for a twenty-minute walk on the apartment balcony's fifty-foot length. A power walk is what I'm aiming for, but it doesn't start that way. First there's the plodding-along stage, which slowly advances to an amiable amble, then to a pretty decent stroll, until finally it becomes what more closely resembles a real walk, admittedly short of a true power walk, but I can feel my steps becoming more powerful as I rack up the miles, and that's strength enough for me at this time.

The walk covers so many backs and forths, I can recite how many pickets line the condo railing, how many aberrations exist in the concrete, and how many steps it takes to cover half a mile.

I must resemble an old, caged animal, pacing in its cage, eyeing freedom just inches away, yet too defanged and scrawny to even consider escaping.

To relieve the ennui exercise induces, I engage in philosophical chats with Rover about the nature of healing, who's going to win the French Open, and whether the breasts of the woman in the swimming pool are hers or silicone-assisted. Rover is mostly silent during these discussions, except for when he makes sloshing sounds to alert me to walk him to the toilet. He knows nothing about tennis, cares less about the inner structure of a woman's mammary glands, but when it comes to healing, his silence is just the ticket. It forces me to consider the unalterable fact that I can't rush the healing process, that it will take as long as it has to, and that I better damn well get used to it. Vague, yes, but on the money for a dog. Good old Rover. Man without a prostate's best friend.

Our cats are another story. They stare at me as if I had just descended from an alien spacecraft, an outerspace creature toting a squiggly, plastic life-support system, designed specifically to frighten felines. Or is it the odor of urine that puts them off? Who wouldn't be put off knowing someone perched a lot higher on the evolutionary scale is peeing in a bag. Cats may be dumb, but they're not stupid, which is how I'm beginning to feel. *Did I do the right thing? Should I have waited instead of rushing into things? Was it a big mistake not getting a second opinion? Could I have learned more?* Damned second thoughts muddy my confidence. Here it is, less than a week after the operation, and I'm a Monday morning quarterback tsk-tsking all the calls, this, in spite of the fact that it's late to call in another coach, or change the game plan now that the ball is in play.

Phone calls from friends and relatives aren't much help, well-intentioned or not. Everybody has well-meaning and, probably, sound advice, but they have no words capable of wishing away my despondent mood. In the end, I wind up consoling them.

Rose understands. She allows me a few calls at first, figuring a talk with friends will buoy me up, but after realizing these conversations seem to depress me even more, they're cut off. She tells everybody I am sleeping, which is not a lie, since napping has become a way of life. Only one person is permitted to connect with me at any time: Tommy. His words, she knows, will be balm for my injured spirits. With him, there will be no platitudes about how well I sound, no false reassurances that I'm going to be okay, no treading lightly over rough ground. Tommy cuts to the tough stuff without flinching. He draws me out, allowing me to voice my every pain and fear, give vent to all my confusion and misgivings, then puts all my woes into a rational perspective, calming the storm of emotions that threaten to capsize my mental boat. Tommy also does what no one else seems to be able to do these days—not Rose, not Imus, not even George Carlin. He makes me laugh so hard, I find myself begging him to stop lest a stitch break apart. From almost 3,000 miles away, he heals me with his friendship, medicine you can't get at a pharmacy.

The thought of work, or the lack of it, hadn't crossed my mind (or bothered me, for that matter) since well before the operation, so wrapped up have I been with my physical concerns. As a free-lancer, you get used to ignoring the wallows, which are oftimes long, but always temporary, the feast or famine syndrome consultants learn to live with.

Rose has admonished me not to answer the phone, to let the answering machine do the work, but while she's out, I can't resist and pick up a call. It's Mel, with a job for me.

"Can you handle it?" he asks.

An assignment would reassure me that even though I'm out of it, I can still function and produce as if I were whole.

"Of course I can handle it," I lie. "I didn't have brain surgery!"

"Are you sure?" A last chance to change my mind, or at least come clean.

I hold fast, so he plugs me into the basic nature of the product, the target audience, everything I'll need to know to complete the job.

"What's the time frame, Melvin?"

"Well . . . we're seeing the client tomorrow afternoon—"

"You'll get it, you bozo. Only next time, why don't you call me at the last fucking minute!"

I hang up while Mel is still laughing, and begin to contemplate my notes.

The product is an umbrella with a unique selling proposition: it won't turn inside out, even in a gale wind. Wind tunnel tests performed in an Air Force facility prove it works. I have to name it, describe its virtues, and in so doing, convince the world they must have this breakthrough brolly. I dub it "The Un-Brella."

What should have been a fun task, turns out to be a torture. Trying to write in bed is about as enjoyable as having root canal work and I wind up having to use the top of the piano as a desk. Sitting comfortably is obviously still to come.

After what seems like three lifetimes, not three weeks, July sixteenth arrives, a sunny, looked-forward-to, tingling with anticipation, emancipation-from-the-catheter day. I can picture, as we drive into Tampa, how wonderful it will feel not to be shackled to a plastic bag.

Sorry, Rover, old fella. But truth is, in spite of our conversations, you didn't bring a helluva lot to the table, and it sure wasn't nice knowing you. So no regrets, erstwhile pal. Hope I won't be seeing you again.

I can also picture the leg catheter bag filling up.

My first post-operative checkup is not with Doctor Tom, who is on vacation, but with his assistant surgeon, Leffie Carlton III.

I'd met Carltons before, but never a third, and especially not a Leffie. I'm intrigued. When he enters the examining room, before he takes my hand he feigns peeking inside my trousers. "Ah, now I remember you!" he says, his good humor and obvious confidence a gift.

After introducing Rose, and since the visit has started on such an up note, I chance what might be an inappropriate question. "Doctor Carlton? Your first name. I've never come across it. If it's not out of line, may I ask where it derives from?"

He generously explains that it's a pet name, a shortened version of Lafayette, a first name that was popular way back when, but which has lost its top ten status as a boy's name long ago. Of course! Add a whiff of the old South and Laffy morphs into Leffie effortlessly.

On the examining table, pants around my knees, Doctor Carlton unceremoniously cuts the catheter tube in half, leaving about three inches of tubing dangling from my penis. The plastic bag and the remaining tubing are thrown in the trash. All that remains is to remove the catheter. With one hand, he holds my penis, with the other he begins to pull gently on the remaining tubing. Another gentle pull.

And again. Now a mild tug. It seems the catheter isn't coming out. This can't be happening. The catheter tube is dripping urine all over the place, raining on my parade. Sweat, mine, adds to the deluge. The back of my legs, needless to say, are begging to be scratched. Good Lord.

Doctor Carlton, brow slightly furrowed, offers as how the balloon end of the Foley, the part that keeps the catheter in place, hasn't deflated and, as such, is prevented from coming out. (Here I'd been so insanely careful, fearing the loathsome device might fall out if jiggled too hard.)

"What can be done about it?" I ask, foreseeing a trip to the hospital for some gruesome emergency procedure to divorce me from Mr. Foley. The day, this bright, happy day, has turned into a nightmare.

"Relax, Bert. I haven't lost a patient during a catheter removal, yet. I'll be back with a wire. It'll be just fine."

I look at Rose. "A wire?" She shrugs. Normally, she's the coach, full of false encouragement. Not today. Not this pissy, stressful, gloomy day that never should have started in the first place. Doctor Carlton is soon back with what resembles a miniature Roto-Rooter: a lengthy coil of wire, ending in a sharp tip.

My intestines are shrinking back, desperately trying to hide behind me as he approaches.Slowly and ever so gently, he begins to slide the tip of the wire into the catheter tube. My heart has traveled into my throat; breathing is impossible.

A sudden, sharp sting in my bladder forces my nervous system into crying, "ouch!"My mouth follows suit.

"Good. I think we burst the balloon," says the doctor, in his I've-got-everything-under-control manner. With that, he slowly withdraws the wire from the tube and sets it aside. And again, holding my penis in one hand, he gingerly wiggles and pulls at the tube and, miraculously, the catheter slides out. Relief is immediate and immense, close to orgasmic.

"You can get dressed now," Doctor Carlton offers as he discreetly leaves the room. Nicest words I ever heard.

The sun is shining again. Putting on diapers for the first time dims its gleam a bit, but for the moment, having said goodbye to Rover makes the day.

Daybook Entry, 6/16/94
(per Dr. Carlton, assistant surgeon)

Patient: Bert Gottlieb

Status post radical prostatectomy: *Patient doing well. Wound clean and dry, with no evidence of infection.*

Catheter removal: *Cut the balloon port off, water came out, however, the catheter didn't, though there was no pain when pulled. Balloon must not have been sufficiently deflated. A .035 guide wire was put up through the balloon port and broke the balloon, allowing the catheter to be removed easily.*

Patient is on Trimethoprim 100 mg. bid, to be continued for 5 more days.

Patient is to schedule a follow-up appointment in 2 weeks with Dr. Mawn.

By the time we get home from a celebratory dinner at, of course, Rio Bravo, the Margaritas have had their way with my open drainage system, and I'm in sore need of a diaper change, my first solo flight into the rituals of incontinence. Where's a mother when you need her?

The front two straps are unbuttoned first. Then you have to catch the diaper before it falls. Next comes undoing the remaining back buttons, deep-sixing the old diaper, buttoning the straps into the back of the fresh diaper, positioning it, buttoning the front straps, then, at long last, pulling it up. Nothing to it once you've learned how to keep the straps untangled.

As recuperative therapy, Rose has brought home a replacement for Rover, an orange and white Scottish Fold kitten named Bitsy (formal name: Elizabeth, Queen of Scotland), who delights in playing with the diaper straps, knocking them out of my hands, dragging out an already overlong bathroom visit even further. In spite of that, she is a precious diversion, and now that I'm home full-time, she'll be the first critter to come into our household I'll be able to bond with and, naturally, spoil a little. Okay, a lot.

Over vitamins, massage therapies, whatever alternate approach there is, give me a kitten anyday.

Short trips to the market, my only outings, require filling my fanny pack with fresh diapers, just in case. Once there, I can't concentrate on shopping, or wait to get home, so focused am I on my condition. No matter that I tell myself no one can see that I'm wearing diapers, let alone see through slacks, I am acutely aware of and uneasy with them, because I constantly feel the hot discharge of urine and don't yet know how much can be absorbed by the diaper, or how much time it will take. I'm good for two aisles and then I'm off to the restroom to check for leakage.

Rose, ever the paragon of patience, understands and, saint that she is, doesn't load the wagon with impulse items while I'm busy checking the load capacity of Depends. Unfortunately, once we're shopped, I have to wait in the car while she endures the checkout line, fretting there isn't a credit card I can use to top up my personal energy levels with.

Diaper days; damp realities. Diaper nights; wet dreams. Childlike before my time, I am wetting incessantly. I can't step out of the shower without putting a diaper on, lest I dribble all over. Yet no matter how careful I am, I leave tracks. A urethral burning, indicating

131

a possible something or other, shows me just how many.

Over the phone, Doctor Carlton prescribes AZO Standard, an over-the-counter treatment for minor urinary infections.

In a few days, the burning is gone, but since the medication turns urine a vivid orange, my pecker tracks—normally the color of lager beer and barely discernible—now are visible on the floor, the mat, the bowl, the seat, the towel, my briefs and my favorite bathrobe. My world is awash in a sea of bright orange dots. While I clean them up, I tell myself to look on the bright side, but the neon glow of reality blinds me from seeing things clearly.

Rose and I finally give up calling them diapers. It had seemed right at the start; defiant, unflinching in the face of adversity, very adult. But the word, not to mention the brave facade, quickly palled and crumbled. Which led to the conundrum of what to call something you have to talk about all the time, but hate its name. "Things" are too vague and inelegant. "Depends," their real name? Not unless there's an advertising allowance forthcoming from the company. (Depending on where they're shopped, a big bag, which lasts maybe five, six days, costs around eighteen dollars, and is not covered by medical insurance or deductible from taxes. I'd switched from the less expensive, button strap model to the pricier velcro strap type after the first bag, since it speeded up the changing process, but unfortunately diminished Bitsy's fun.)

Still, the question of what to call a diaper other than a diaper begged for an answer. *How about "G-string"? I don't think so. "Loincloth"? Much too Tarzan. Does "dydee" do anything for you? Of course: it makes caca.*

We obviously needed a word that said "diaper" and yet didn't, a word that sort of mimicked it, yet with a more whimsical, possibly enigmatic twist.

The answer comes to us from a Britcom on PBS. *Nappies!*

Short for napkins. A little babyish and somewhat arcane, but if that's what the Brits call them, and since we're closet Anglophiles, why not. So nappies they become, though diapers they remain.

Bloody hell.

For Father's Day, my son and daughter-in-law have planned a barbecue party which I am duty-bound to attend. This first social outing fills me with dread, but I know how important it is for my kids to see me up and about. I can't blame them, and I can't disappointment them or their friends, who have also become my friends.

The day is fresh and bright, the food equally so, and the company so warm, I don't think about my condition. It is so good to be talking with everyone and cooking alongside my son, I forget about the nappie situation. For hours, I'm blissfully inattentive to anything but this rare, special time, with all of us gabbing away, nibbling and drinking, enjoying each other immensely. Then it comes to me that I haven't checked myself in quite a while. I get up to leave the table and my hand happens to rub across the back of my shorts. I am wet, and about ten levels above mortified, even though I'm the only one aware of my predicament.

In the guest john, I change myself and do my best to blot my shorts dry, but they remain damp enough to tell the tale. From the kitchen, I beckon Rose off the porch.

"What's the matter?"

I point to the back of my shorts.

"So you're a little wet. No one'll notice."

"Except me. Please, let's go home," I beg and demand. Rose knows better than to argue. She says goodbye to everyone, explaining our sudden departure with a white lie about my having to be back in bed; actually, it's half the truth.

David I tell the truth to. We are as much brothers as we are father and son and have always shared the good and the bad stuff.

"I could have loaned you a pair of shorts, Dad."

"I know, sweetheart, but . . . " I stare at the ground, wanting to crawl into it.

"Hey. That's okay. Leave your only son without a father on Father's Day. See if I care." He smiles the smile that can light up the dark. He hugs me. He understands.

For my second post-op visit—this time with Doctor Tom—I fuss at my toilet more than usual. I want to look my best for him; a small offering of a patient's appreciation; a way of saying, "See what a good job you did!" Or maybe it's because I am feeling better—not strong enough yet, certainly not dry enough, but better—and that's worth the extra effort.

Tom, after a series of gentle pokes and questions, patiently listens to me describe the way my incontinence works, as if he's not heard the same tale hundreds of times before.

Lying down or sitting, I explain, there is little, if any, leakage. But once up, I can feel myself starting to urinate. Thanks to Mr. Kegel, I'm able to control some of the flow, allowing me enough time to reach the toilet. But the sphincter isn't always strong enough. *So it's an unwinnable battle. Gravity wins each skirmish for the bathroom high ground. Try as you might, want as much as you want, you are powerless against your angry and injured flesh. This is the price you paid to live free from cancer. These are the wounds you knew you might incur when you joined up. Get used to it, soldier. This is the way it's gonna be until continence returns. And when and if it it does, as it will for ninety-percent of you grunts, it will do so in its own good time, which can vary any where from a couple of weeks to a couple of years; it's different for each man. Until then, dogface, remember who's in charge.*

"Give it time, Bert. You're doing fine." Doctor Tom, playing Coach Mawn, brings me back to earth. I hear what he's saying, and

I so want to believe him.

Daybook Entry 7/1/94

<u>Patient:</u> *Bert Gottlieb*

<u>Reason for visit:</u> *Post-op checkup five weeks after radical. Catheter was removed on the third post-operative week, not without a struggle, I see from Leffie's notes. Today's urinalysis reveals many white blood cells; will culture. Currently not on antibiotics. There appears to be some gain in continence at night, but none during the day. Return visit in 1 month.*

<u>Post Visit Thoughts & Observations:</u> *The regaining of continence generally follows three stages: first, dry lying down (at night); then, dry walking around; and lastly, dry when standing up after sitting. Bert, obviously, is still in the first stage. His impatience is not atypical. I can only imagine how frustrating this has to be for him. It is frustrating, too, for the physician, since the best and only advice he can offer is to have patience, that the odds are for continence to return, with the understanding that it won't return all at once. That said, I am impatient for him to get past this upsetting period.* In the month before my next visit, I have the opportunity to talk with two men about their prostate cancer experiences. One makes me feel smart, the other that I've become an expert on the subject.

Conversation with the first man, a vague acquaintance whom I judge to be in his mid-to-late sixties, starts innocently with his asking after my health, post radical surgery.

I, of course, tell him everything, permission to be boring being the absolute right of a prostate cancer survivor.

"Some of those things you talked about . . . the scores, staging . . . I just went along with my doctor . . . maybe I shouldn't have . . . I don't know . . . " And he starts to cry.

I'm sorry I ever said anything.

"Were you left incontinent like me?" I ask, figuring it might be consoling if he believed I was in the same boat.

"No, I have no problems that way."

"Well, that's good. How about erections?"

Through clenched teeth, he whispers, "I'm psychologically impotent!"

I could kick myself; I didn't want to share his depressing secret. "If you're sure it's not physical, maybe a chat with a—"

"I'm not chatting with anybody. I'm just angry with my doctor."

The story is, he just washed his hands of any responsibility, the ignorance is bliss strategy. He had no idea of his PSA levels pre- or post-surgery, never heard of, or bothered to find out about Gleason scores or staging procedures, couldn't recall any pre-operative tests, didn't speak to a radiotherapist or any other qualified clinician, and hadn't seen his doctor since his catheter was removed four years ago.

"Are you sure you had a radical?" I ask, figuring he might have had a TURP.* instead, and lacking even rudimentary knowledge, was somehow confused.

"I'm not sure of anything," he answers dejectedly.

He can't remember if the DRE revealed any irregularities, or whether it was BPH symptoms which had initiated the subsequent procedures, or even what the procedures were. He took a journey on faith, never questioning why it was heading where it was, what the fare was, when he would arrive, or what he would be like when he got to his destination, and now he's shattered, his fury barely contained.

"Maybe you should sit down with your doctor and tell him how you feel . . . ask some questions . . . it might clear things up."

---

*A Transurethral Resection Procedure (or TURP) improves BPH problems quickly. With an instrument called a resectoscope inserted in the penis, the tissue blockage is removed, unclogging the urethral pipes, so to speak.

"Me, talk to that sonofabitch?"

No, I thought, let your anger eat away at you as if it were a cancer. It was easy feeling smarter than him, difficult feeling sorry.

My second conversation is with the father of a young woman I know. He tells me he is a hale sixty years of age, post radical, post catheter by a few weeks, worried that he hasn't dried up yet, and what do I think? First, I give him the third degree: PSA, DRE results, Gleason score, staging numbers, pre-op test results, the works. He has all the answers. I remind him of how great the odds are in favor of his regaining continence, but that it's gonna take its own sweet time to return, so he should relax and just go about his life.

"You sound like my doctor," he says.

"Then listen to your doctor, my friend."

Here was a man who worked with his hands, not a white collar employee like the first man I spoke with, yet this simple man managed to learn enough about his condition to make an informed decision. From everything he told me, I believed his urologist had guided him surely and professionally through the process, which thought had me wondering just when I felt I knew enough about prostate cancer matters to pass judgment on a physician's performance.

That qualm aside, it felt good to help someone, even if help was just a good ear, another veteran you could rehash war stories with, someone who could remind you that, no matter what the scars, the bloody fight was worth it.

As an incontinent, stage one actor, I made a good preacher, but a lousy congregation member. Maybe in time I'd believe my own lines.

* * *

Chapter 8
Still No Cigar

The month of July sees me walking a few miles every other day, my weight coming back on, the psoriasis (or whatever the hell it is) under control, the rash on my back long gone, and the family jewels looking brighter. I should be delighted, but waiting for the post-operative PSA test, worrying whether it will bless or damn the decision to proceeed as we did, dulls any enjoyment I might have taken in my healing body. Knowing the odds are in my favor isn't good enough; I have to hear the fat lady sing. I may or may not have lost the pissing contest, but I must know if I won the goddamned war. Until I receive good news from the front, I'll hold off doing my George C. Scott General Patton imitation.

Despite the crotchets, life is returning to normal—slower than I'd like, but heading in the right direction. So why am I so down in the dumps?

Doctor Tom tells me I look great, considering it's been only two months since my surgery. I must be getting good at keeping a lid on my depression. Either that, or he's a good liar.

My third post-op visit and it's a sullen replay of the last one: same inspection, same incontinence stage.

I have to keep reminding myself that healing is a process and that I must learn to go with its flow or risk banging my head against the wall, as my old friend Ziggy would mix the metaphor. My concerns have me off-balance and I can't seem to keep from tripping no matter how hard I try to shake them.

Tom's smiles and reassurances are not much help, either.

Daybook Entry 8/1/94

Patient: Bert Gottlieb

Reason for visit: *Post-op checkup 9 weeks after radical. Incision is healing well. Some continence at night, none during the day. Urine still presents numerous white and red blood cells. Will repeat urine culture. Return visit in two months, with PSA test prior to visit.*

Post Visit Thoughts & Observations: *Physically, Bert is on schedule, if not ahead of it. His post partum funk, which he tries to hide, is not unusual, and I'm confident he'll pull out of it once he's gained back more energy and passed his next hurdle—the first post-op PSA test.*

It happened. I blew my next appointment with Doctor Tom, having had the blood test a week prior, and obviously didn't find out my PSA results.

How it happened is I pasted the bright, yellow reminder sticker on the wrong page of the calendar. The next visit is rescheduled thirty cloudy days ahead.

For close to four months I've been anticipating each day would be the day the urine died, the day I could stop checking my horoscope for signs of imminent success in matters of health, the moment I could uncross my fingers.

Being rejected *by* your body is almost worse than being rejected *for* it. The inability to handle rejection is what kept me from pursuing an acting career. My first and only open call for a Broadway show lasted as long as it took to recite my name before being hustled into the street by an assistant stage manager. Never had my ego felt so battered. Was I too short, too thin, too blonde, too what? They could have said something besides "Thank you!"

And yet, forty years later, I get up each morning eager to be acting some part other than that of a cripple, but before I can even think of my name I have to check my diaper for yet another rejection. After this, Broadway begins to look easy. As I work at keeping the velcro straps from sticking to each other, I hear myself aping Rod Serling: ... *doomed to trod the boards for eternity, Mr. Gottlieb doesn't realize yet ... that he's never getting past Stage One ... that he'll be forever wondering why he didn't get the part of the long lost lover. He doesn't know he's entered ... The Diaper Zone. DEE-dah-DEE-dah. DEE-dah-DEE-dah.*

The big day. The candles are lit.

"What's my number, Tom?" I ask before we've even finished shaking hands.

"Zero point five," he answers with a big smile.

I passed the test! I'm not going to flunk out! Zero point five! What a lovely number! Were there ever three more beautiful words, a more dizzying thought?

I am brought back to earth by Tom donning a rubber glove and asking me to assume the position.

Over my shoulder, I ask, "Why, if I have no prostate anymore, are you poking around up there?"—quickly adding, because I am giddy at being able to breathe again, and because I realize Tom's had to have been asked this question too many times before—"Or is it love?"

"You want the clinical spiel, or the simple explanation?"

"As long as it doesn't include a proposition, take your pick."

"Simple it is then," Tom continues, his grin still intact. "What I'm doing is checking to see that the prostatic area of concern to me is healing as it should."

"And is it?"

"Yes, it is, Bert, and so are you. Go out and celebrate tonight with Rose."

"I will. And Tom—I know I've said it before, but thanks."

"Get outta here, I've got sick people to see."

Daybook Entry 11/30/94

<u>Patient:</u> Bert Gottlieb
<u>Reason for Visit:</u> 6 month post-op checkup
<u>PSA</u>: 0.5 Ng/Ml
<u>DRE:</u> Revealed no induration of the prostatic fossa.
<u>Urinalysis:</u> Positive improvement, virtually normal, some bacterial presence.
<u>Observations:</u> Voiding freely, still incontinent, though dry at night. Otherwise, he is markedly better than he was at his last visit, able to function quite well inside and out of the house, and was obviously pleased and relieved to hear his low PSA number, as was I.
Return visit in 3 months, PSA prior. Letter to Dr. Dominguez.

Unlike Eliot's Prufrock, I measure out my days in diapers rather than coffee spoons. My crotch controls my life. Do I need a change yet? Can I stretch the one I'm wearing for another hour? Are the back of my pants okay? Do I dare to eat a peach? Prufrock was right about the mermaids: I do not think that they will sing to me, especially since I live mainly in my bathroom, surrounded by books, magazines, crossword puzzles, nappie straps, changes of underwear, and the pissiest of moods.

A hermit is what I've become. And I feel like a shit because I know how it impacts on Rose, how turning down invitations is killing her. A loner by choice, incontinence provides me with the best excuse for my seeming aloofness and my inability to handle small talk for more than a few minutes, while it robs Rose of the nourishment I alone can't provide for her.

Even when she can persuade me into going out, I'm not what you'd call an ideal guest. I smile and I chat, but my mind is always on my trouser's inseam, calculating rates of flow and absorption, the diuretic affects of alcohol and caffeine, and whether black jeans can truly hide a damp patch. When you're on diaper duty, far from the safety of home, you cannot let your mind wander lest you drop your defenses and wind up saying goodnight, while sidestepping with your back against the wall as you head toward the front door.

Thanksgiving and Christmas celebrations at our house are as expected: I'm as juicy as the turkey.

This was the first New Year's Eve I ever looked forward to. The past year was not a vintage year, one to be savored and lingered over. It was a watershed year, though, the dividing point between life with cancer and life with hope.

When Times Square erupts, ushering in '95, it brings with it, not just the joy of saying goodbye (and good riddance) to a year best forgotten, but an unusual and unexpected occurrence: an erection. It is an achy one, and not as an old southern friend once described it: "So hard a cat couldn't scratch it!" But it was solid enough proof that the nerve bundles that control erectile function had been spared.

Rose and I toast Tom Mawn and make a resolution never to buy a wine bottled in '94.

Although having sex in my leaky state was a non-starter, the thought had crossed my mind. So did the question of when. Assuming I regained continence, when would I, let alone my still tender penis, know when it was okay to resume sex?

My friend Mel had the answer. He told me what his doctor had said to a friend of his who'd been circumcised late in life and who wanted to know when he could safely go back to making love. The sage medical advice: "When the ecstacy exceeds the agony."

I couldn't think of a better motto, nor a more hopeful start to the New Year than this erection, a sign that maybe, just maybe, everything was going to be all right after all.

What a propitious start for '95. For the first time in my life, I make a resolution: try and get out more.

We're not into the new year but two months, and my resolution—an iffy pledge at best—goes the way of all champagne promises.

It's the second post-op PSA and it's the same wonderful low number, so it's off to Rio Bravo for a rare night out.

The chips and salsa, the beer, and our good (so far) fortune, declare it a celebration.

As we contemplate the entree selections, I begin to cough, nailed by an overly-zealous jalapeno, loosing a stressed stream of urine, enough to overburden the nappy and make me extremely uncomfortable. Trouper that I am, I don't call attention to the accident until after dinner. Rose hurts for me, and with not a gripe, bitch or grumble, she accepts my discomfort, disappointment and embarrassment as hers. If I can't go out, neither will she. Shipmates for close to thirty-five years, we'll just tack in a different direction until the weather clears. No big deal as long as we're on this voyage together.

A consistent stream of work from two agencies in New York, and an assortment of local assignments, provides needed distraction, as does the O.J. trial, without which I couldn't have made it through the year. I was so addicted to this judicial entertainment, the personalities of its players, and its fascinating (albeit mind-numbing) quasi-scientific presentations, I was able to think about nothing else. While I urged Christopher Darden to speed up his delivery, I was focused only on Judge Ito's courtroom and the shenanigans of the attorneys. What a mindless feast for stay-at-homes—especially the chronically wet.

Two events conspire to make '95 a better year than we bargained for. One is a medical miracle, the other is a miracle of the heart.

The medical miracle is urged on by Rose who, having watched me struggle with my skin condition (and, being Rose, suffering along with me), has had it with the psoriasis diagnosis.

Medical text out, she spreads the dermatological color plates before me.

"Okay, poster boy. It's been over a year. Look at all these pretty pictures and tell me what you think you've got now."

This is it: high noon at the not-so-o.k. corral.

I hitch up my velcro straps and stare long and hard at the pictures, then at Rose, who is standing there, hands on her hips, ready to gun me down if I make a wrong move.

"Well, ma'am, you were right. It sure don't look like psoriasis—unless of course, it takes longer to become crusty and icky like in them pictures there."

Rose raises an eyebrow.

"All right. It's not psoriasis. But what the hell is it, then?"

She uncocks her 44's. Phew. I was out of ammunition.

"I'd say it's either this or this," Rose says, pointing to "eczema" and then to "shingles."

We decide in favor of eczema, since there was never any pain, a major shingles sympton.

"But I don't know another dermatol . . ."

"Here's the number of a well-respected one in St. Pete. Call her tomorrow."

"Yes, ma'am." I hate shootouts.

Doctor Talley, a dermatologist at Bayfront Medical Center, couldn't be more professional.   Eczema is, of course, her diagnosis. No scrapings. No doubts. And the amazing thing is, I believe her.

"But what could have caused it?"

"Many things. Detergents, allergies . . . hard to say."

"How about stress?"

"What do you call stress?"

"Well, my daughter's just become engaged and we're preparing for her wedding."

"That could be stressful, but that's a good kind of stress."

"How about a radical prostatectomy?" I saved the best for last.

"Now that would be stressful. Your eczema could, indeed, then, be due to internal pressures."

"So what's the cure? Ten milligrams of Valium and a bunch of hours on the couch?"

"No," she laughs. "A prescription for a steroid cream to quell the itching and—much as I'm sure you'll hate it—a twenty minute soak in a colloidal oatmeal bath every day, after which you'll apply a special moisturizer."

She was right: I detest baths. But I promise to follow through.

Her last words to me, as she flies off to another patient, are, "Relax. Enjoy your daughter's wedding."

Dermatologist and psychologist, no extra charge.

The second miracle is my daughter's wedding, which requires traveling to New Jersey twice: once, to meet the in-laws to be, and to attend the engagement party; then the actual wedding.

My daughter's new family is as down to earth and quirky as ours; a perfect fit. Most important, they've unconditionally welcomed Lori into their family, showering her with love and grace. And if we had asked for another son, Lori's husband-to-be would have been it.

New Jersey didn't cure any of my hermit-like symptoms. I found that if I cocooned in the hotel all day, I could endure dinner out or a family get together.

By now, I was much better at calculating my output versus the overflow potential of the nappies, and as long as I had a ready supply of them, I could relax somewhat. To feel really at ease, I had to be in the hotel room, out of the spotlight I irrationally felt was trained on me. In the hotel room, I was an anonymous body, a dry voice on the phone talking to friends, making up apologies for not being able to see them this time around, safe from the accident that was ever waiting to happen. (I used the wedding preparations as my excuse, even though it was Rose who was out with Lori all day on a mother-daughter shopathon, while I lolled around the "house" in my robe.)

Strangely, I wasn't reluctant to talk to people about my condition, but there was no way I could begin to explain how I felt when I was out of the nest, the constant buzz of disquiet, how a part of my brain was always fixated on on my goddamned condition, no matter where I was, or whom I was talking with. If agoraphobia is an abnormal fear of being in a public place, what's the Greek word for fear of peeing in a public place?

That aside, this first trip to Bergen County in years, was a real up for me, thanks to Lori Joy's good fortune to meet Mr. Right, a wonder in this day and age.

There's something about a wedding that blurs the perceptions; everything is too fast, too much, too wonderful to recall anything but the highlights: carefully stuffing my tuxedo pockets with nappies, making sure they didn't bulge out and give themselves away; standing opposite my daughter, moments before heading down the aisle, she and I doing our best not to cry, and mostly succeeding, since one of the mottoes in our house has been "the show must go on;" surreptitiously dabbing at my eyes during the excruciatingly-long Lutheran ceremony (I say that about all wedding ceremonies regardless of denomination.), and being caught at it by Rose who, in sign language, tells everyone around us; seeing Mel and Sol after so long a time, and sharing this extraordinary time with them; that very special moment the bride danced with her father and cried in his arms, daddy's little girl no more; enjoying the food and the impeccable service, courtesy of me, with everything as promised by the Banquet Manager, thanks to his having a thing for Mrs. Gutt-leeb, and so eager to please and gain favor in his blonde goddess' eyes, he made sure every oily promise was kept; saying goodbye to old friends; partying until the wee hours with the bride and groom and their friends in the bride and groom's room, and bouncing up the next morning to have breakfast with the kids and the friends that had survived the after-wedding affair; all that I remember, and shall never forget.

My daughter's wedding was proof that with enough excitement, including stress, and you can almost live with the bad stuff.

My third post-op PSA test result in June of '95 is the same as the last one: continued good news. Other than the perpetual drip, I appear to be doing fine. Doctor and patient both seem to be past heightened concern and can only shuffle their feet and agree that perhaps a little more time has to pass before writing off continence comeback. At least visits will be every six months from now on; a longer leash on life.

Although the checkup has by now become a perfunctory ritual, it is always encouraging to see Tom.

Daybook Entry 6/2/95

Patient: *BG*
Reason for visit: *9 month post-op checkup*
PSA: *0.5 Ng/Ml*
DRE: *No induration of the postatic fossa.: Normal*
Urinalysis: Normal
Return visit in 6 months, PSA prior.
Post Visit Thoughts & Observations: Urinary incontinence continues, with patient dry at night and somewhat dryer during the day than he's been. Bert's spirits and his energy level seem to be

much higher than they were at the last visit. His daughter got married a few weeks ago, and he seems not only to have survived the ordeal, but thrived on it. I hope this is the beginning of what has been a painfully slow recovery cycle.

The year was not without medical incident.

Another part of my anatomy, my shoulder, decided to enliven the remainder of the year. It had been bothering me on and off since before the prostate was a problem, but had become so chronically severe, I had to seek help from a specialist, a bone doctor Rose had been to once, and who seemed proficient enough, she thought, to handle a shoulder. The doctor—young, pleasant, slick—not only told me I needed an operation on my shoulder, but went about setting it up with alarming speed. Yellow alert.

He used the X-ray of my shoulder to buttress his decision to rush into surgery. Unfortunately, the picture he showed me resembled nothing like the bone structure of any shoulder I'd ever seen in any anatomical text. Calling a white dot on a black field an encroaching bursa, does not a clavicle or a scapula make. Second yellow alert.

When I conveyed my fear that something done to the shoulder might possibly affect my hands, he pooh-poohed my concern. Even after I made it clear that in my work and my life I needed my hands, used them daily on two keyboards—piano and computer—both of which required not only the full compliment of digits, but complete cooperation from the shoulder—he maintained that after two months of therapy I'd be practically new. Red alert.

Since I knew no other shoulder specialists, I did the next best thing: called a foot doctor I was friendly with, figuring he would know a good bone man. He did. He also was acquainted with the procedure I was being asked to undergo, but had seen too many foreshortened arms with limited articulation to put his blessings on a shoulder operation which, if memory serves, he called a Gleason (shades of the prostate go-around) Procedure . Instead, he gave me the name of a first-rate orthopedic surgeon who, after re-X-raying my shoulder (his pictures looked as if they came out of a textbook), recommended therapy as the first course of action, and only if that failed, which he sincerely doubted, might he then consider arthroscopy. He agreed with me that hands, when stretched out, should, if at all possible, be the same length and equally as strong.

After six weeks of hot packs, ultra sound, and pressure and weight exercises, the shoulder was almost back to normal.

Sometime during the therapy sessions my chiropodist friend informed me that in checking around, he had found out that Dr. Hurry-Up-And-Chop had an expensive lifestyle to maintain, and my shoulder probably would have paid the leases on his two new Lexi.

Once again, my instincts didn't let me down, though this time they demanded a second opinion.

On balance, the pluses of '95 outweighed the minuses.

"Here's to a dry '96," Rose toasts.

"Yeah," I answer flatly.

"Could we have a touch more enthusiasm?!"

"Yeah, yeah."

"Kiss me, you jerk."

We fall asleep holding hands before Guy Lombardo drowns us in treacle, vowing before we nod off, to celebrate a new year in our own very good time

* * *

Chapter 9

Life Membership

It's been over a year and a half since the operation and I'm not yet fully recovered. I expected more, wanted not just something, but everything to be all right. Knowing it could have been a helluva lot worse isn't enough, but it does dole out a measure of guilt, ever the leavening agent. I made it so far, how dare I whine over spilled urine? Isn't being cancer-free enough? It should be, and I should be ashamed, for there are far greater personal afflictions than incontinence. You can live with incontinence.

There's this two-man sweat shop somewhere in the bowels of New York City's Garment Center. The Cutter stands on one side of the meager workbench, scissoring fabric yard after interminable yard. The Sewer sits cross-legged atop his side of the workbench, carefully placing the needle into the fabric, then pulling it out to somewhere near his cheek, repeating this universal motion over and ever over. Forty-five years of this brainless concentration has taken its toll on conversation, their words worn out years ago. Now they only talk.

CUTTER: So where you going on your vacation?

SEWER (TEARING A KNOT OFF WITH HIS TEETH): Africa.

CUTTER: So what are you going to do in Africa?

SEWER (TAKING A FEW STITCHES): Hunt lions.

CUTTER: So what do you know about hunting lions?

SEWER: What I don't know, I'll learn.

A month passes and the Sewer is atop his workbench, back at work.

CUTTER: So how was Africa?

SEWER (PULLING OUT A BAD STITCH BEFORE ANSWERING): Not bad.

CUTTER: Did you find any lions?

SEWER: Of course, I found lions.

CUTTER: Did you kill any lions?

SEWER: No, but a lion killed me.

CUTTER: If a lion killed you, Mr. Smartie World Traveler, how come you're still alive?

SEWER (PAUSING TO BITE OFF A THREAD): You call this living?

In spite of my low expectations, today's visit to the doctor takes a turn upward, albeit in an unexpected direction.

After Tom's DRE, an excellent 0.2 PSA result, and my no-good-news-to- report from the diaper front, I remind myself to tell him, since it might be relevant, that not only have I experienced adequate erections, but an orgasm, as well, retrograde though it may have been. When I get less of a positive reaction than I expected, it hits me: what good is an erection if you can't really use it?

Tom is shaking his head in frustration.

"Bert, we've got to do something about you."

"You mean we shouldn't keep our fingers crossed a little longer?"

"Sorry to say, but it doesn't look like it. If continence was coming back, we would have seen some progress. There's been no change in your condition for more than a year. You're still at Stage One."

"I guess that makes me one of the lucky ten percent."

"There are things that can be done."

I had stopped reading about prostate problems after I'd made my decision to go ahead with surgery. I thought I'd learned enough. Even when boning up on things prostate, I never concentrated on incontinence because I just assumed it wouldn't happen to me, and when it did, assumed again that it would eventually fix itself up. It hasn't. It won't. I'm an eager student again.

"There are collagen injections, but I've not had great success with them. It's an ongoing process, too, not just one set of injections and goodbye. I'm not sure your insurance covers it either. Many companies call it an experimental procedure. Also, any scar tissue from the operation can interfere with the proper placement of the collagen. I just can't recommend it for you."

"Where does that leave us?"

"I have a suggestion. An implant. It does the job your sphincter's not doing."

I wince at the suggestion, but Tom continues. "I don't install it. That's done someplace else. I've read many journal papers on this, attended lectures and seminars on it. Also, two friends, both urologists, have had it done and I've heard no complaints." Tom hands me a videotape. "Before we go any further, watch this. It'll tell you the whole story. Come back in two weeks and we'll talk about it some more."

I can't wait.

Daybook Entry 1/19/96

Patient: BG
Reason for visit: *18 month post-op checkup*
PSA: *0.2 Ng/Ml*
DRE: *No indication of any induration of the prostatic fossa. Return visit in two weeks to discuss implant referral.*
Post Visit Thoughts & Observations: *Today I had to inform*

Bert that his continence did not look like it would return. His gravitational incontinence leaves him with no effective means of control. In spite of excellent internal sphincter control, his external sphincter is helpless to prevent urine from constantly dribbling out. He currently goes through 5 to 6 pads a day.

It is of interest to note that he is having adequate erections and ejaculatory sensation without emission.

I could not recommend collagen treatments for reasons of high cost, modest results (only a small percentage of men stay completely dry), and the fact that post-operative scars can interfere with injections of the collagen, limiting its ability to completely close off the urethra. On top of that, it is an uncomfortable procedure, having oftimes to be repeated until the urethra is fully closed off, or as closed as it will ever be. The process may again have to be repeated a few years down the road as the collagen loses it elasticity and the leakage returns.

I did, however, give him a videotape of a urinary prosthesis that can function in place of his external sphincter, and urged him to watch it. (Actually, I gave him two tapes—one for the sphincter implant, one for the penile prosthesis; I couldn't recall which was which.)

I am eager to see Bert's problem resolved. He tries not to show it, but it's evident in his eyes and the tightly-drawn corners of his mouth that he doesn't seem to be living so much as existing.

For some reason, we didn't get around to looking at the videos right away, the why of which I still don't understand, considering our eagerness to learn more about this possible panacea. It wasn't until the next weekend, after Rose had just made us a brace of impressive BLTs for lunch, that I recalled the videotapes and slipped one into the VCR.

The first one started off well-enough with an executive-type talking head, unctuously presenting the AMS 800 urinary sphincter, a small-enough-to-fit-handily-in-the-palm, solid silicone elastomer, fluid-filled device which, when implanted into the body, can mirror the normal process of urinary control and urination. So far, so good.

The device, it is pointed out, consists of three components: a cuff, a pump and a pressure-regulating balloon, all linked via kink-resistant tubing; a closed-circuit hydraulic pressure machine Rube Goldberg would have envied.

The cuff surrounds the urethra, the balloon goes into the space next to the bladder, and the pump (a roughly 1" x ½" x ¼" plastic, rectangular-shaped piece with soft, curving shoulders at the leading edge) sits in the scrotum. An elegant solution.

The cuff holds the urethra closed. To urinate, the pump is squeezed. This sends the fluid from the balloon (distilled water, I'll presume) into the cuff, opening it. After urinating, the fluid automatically flows back to the balloon, thus closing the urethra and restoring continence again. Pretty neat.

Lecture over, the video cuts to the actual implant procedure with no warning that the film you are about to see may include disturbing material.

Kiss lunch goodbye.

Out of the corner of my eye I peek at the screen, mesmerized, repulsed, awed at the medical and technological ingenuity, pissed that a magnificent sandwich has to go to waste.

Rose, the acknowledged "house ghoul," walks out of the room at the first incision between the scrotum and the anus, muttering, "I can't watch." The video is obviously targeted to clinicians, not civilians. So was the other video, which had as its subject, the penile implant. Curiosity makes me fast foward through it, pausing every so often to watch a few moments in real time. The images of this procedure have me thinking how sort of lucky I am to be incontinent and not impotent and having to decide whether or not to undergo the resurrection of a dead appendage; they don't go away for days.

What the sphincter video did not mention, but which was included in their product literature, were the possible complications, which included *"infection, hematoma, cuff site erosion or atrophy, fluid leak, tubing kink* (sic), *inadequate cuff compression, urethral injury, pump erosion, herniated reservoir and pump malfunction, and other mechanical difficulties."*

But their clinical success rate was high, with close to ninety percent of implanted patients becoming dry or having minimal incontinence. Wonderful. I'm back to another ten percent chance of crapping out and I've lost any stomach I ever had for gambling. With my optimism level registering empty, I couldn't hope to dream for fear of losing again.

Each time I thought about the implant (which was all the time), I envisioned plastic objects jiggling around inside me like toys. I could almost feel their intrusion, the awkwardness they must engender.

On the plus side, I could boast of being a bionic man with an implanted whizzer device made of space-age materials. But would I clunk as I moved? Would the part located in my scrotum swing bell-like against the scrotal walls or the epididimus (ouch) as I walked? If so, would I have to mince to keep everything from jostling around?

Ziggy, I know I can't live without this thing, but I'm not sure I can live with it and, in case you weren't quite sure, I'm scared shitless. Whaddya think?

Ziggy, ever the coward, refuses to commit himself.

The day before we go to see the doctor, I convene a mini-meeting in the supermarket.

"Whatddya think, Ro?"

"The steaks look nice."

"I mean, what do you think about the you-know-what?"

"You don't really have a choice."

"Yes, I do."

"You do?"

"No, I don't . . . I don't know . . . "

"I do. We're having steak."

Meeting adjourned. Motion to proceed with implant tabled for the moment.

"Did you watch the tapes?" is the first question Doctor Tom has.

"I did. Rose couldn't."

"They *are* a bit clinical, but I figured you'd want to know what it was all about before making any kind of decision."

"Why do they have to list all the possible complications?"

Tom reminds me that this prosthesis, though a medical and technological marvel, is still a manufactured product, and all its potential complications must be stated clearly for product liability reasons.

"To cover their ass in case of litigation, in other words." My summation.

"And to give everyone the willies," Rose offers.

"I've heard only good reports about it," Tom hastens to add. I'm outnumbered. Rose stares at me. Her eyes ask, "Well?" I fold. "What's the next step?"

Tom explains that the procedure is performed at the Cleveland Clinic by a Doctor Montague, head of prosthetic surgery, and that he will contact him and start the ball rolling, an apt metaphor as it turned out.

Daybook Entry 2/2/96

Patient: BG
Reason for Visit: Further discussion of external sphincter
implant.
Post Visit Thoughts & Observations: Bert knows he must, and
wants to go ahead, but is apprehensive about the procedure,
which is understandable. His wife encouraged him to do so, as
did I. I have high hopes for his successful recovery.

Daybook Entry 2/3/96
*Followup phone call to Dr. Drogo Montague at Cleveland
Clinic to discuss Bert's situation. Relayed Montague's number
to Bert, who will call him today to make an appointment for
emplacement of the prosthetic sphincter.*

I stare at the unfamiliar name and number for the longest time before
picking up the phone. Reaching out and touching someone who might
be talking to me from a pay phone inside a one-story cinderblock
building is really off-putting.

Reluctantly, I dial the Cleveland number and am informed that
Doctor Montague is on rounds, but will get back to me as soon as he
is through, which he does.

On the phone, the doctor is most cordial and forthright in
answering my questions and adding enough details for me to get the
picture: the implant procedure runs about two and a half hours and
includes an hour of prep; the hospital stay is three days; when re-
leased, you'll still be incontinent until you return six weeks later (everything having had time to heal) to have the pump activated; success
rate is ninety percent, but a pad in your shorts will probably be necessary to absorb the few drops that may escape due to a hard cough or
sneeze; long term results only go back five years; there are two hotels
on campus; you have to be at the Clinic a day before the slated procedure for a full physical, which includes a cystoscope; the Clinic's

insurance people will send you a breakdown of costs and will handle all the paperwork once you're connected; no aspirin two weeks before the procedure date; call Fran to begin the process; looking forward to meeting you.

Before I chicken out by thinking too much, I call the Clinic's eight-hundred number and ask to speak to Fran.

At dinner, Rose asks me if I called Dr. Whatshisname in Cleveland.

I sing "April in Cleveland" to the tune of "April in Paris."

"So you did it, you brave thing! Tell me!"

No sooner do I tell her, than, calendar and pad in lap, she's on the phone chatting with a Missy at Continental making flight arrangements, and then with a Darryl at the Cleveland Omni (which, it turns out, adjoins the clinic) making room reservations.

"Okay." Rose begins as she takes a bite of cold steak. "We leave on a Sunday afternoon . . . have a nice dinner in Cleveland . . . Monday's pre-op day . . . Tuesday the procedure . . . three days in the hospital and we're home on Saturday or Sunday if we have to stay another day."

"I liked the part about the nice dinner."

"It's gonna be fine."

"Tell that to my insides."

"You're gonna be fine," Rose yells at my stomach.

I don't laugh. The pluses and the minuses are still fighting to cancel each other out and come to an agreement. *Maybe you should leave well enough—okay, bad enough— alone. What if your body rejects the implant? It happens. But how nice it will be to be normal again, to ditch the diapers. If everything goes all right, that is. But what could go wrong? Shall we list the ten plus possible complications? C'mon, why shouldn't I get the gold ring this time? Maybe for the same reason you didn't get the golden walnut last time; lucky in love, unlucky in continence. Hell, Tom wouldn't recommend something that wouldn't help. But he doesn't perform the procedure. And you've never even met the guy who does, unless you count a phone call a meeting. You should have gone to Cleveland for a face to face, checked out the facility. What if it is a one-story clinic? They've only been doing this for five years, so it makes you a sort of guinea pig. But go ahead, let them implant their tinker toys (which you never were good at), then everyone can call you Bert, the Bionic Dick. If Ziggy were here, he'd say "you're taking this on faith again and frankly, your belief account is overdrawn, and you haven't made a deposit in who knows how long. Can't say as I blame you, considering how you wound up last time. But you're in it now, kiddo, up to your crotch. How wonderful, though, if it does work."*

Yeah, if.

Everyone has to hear about this, my upcoming adventure into inner space. I need a morale boost from my cheering squad—pats on the back, high fives, the whole go-get-'em-tiger routine.

Al, my brother-in-law, isn't acquainted with implanted prostheses, but offers to send me a medical catalog he's worked on which has an array of leg bags and other external urinary devices, which he claimed did an admirable job, considering. He also wishes me all the luck in the world.

Shellie, who considers a dental checkup invasive surgery, hurts for me, wincing at the thought of my having to undergo another operation, praying with all her fiber that it turns out well.

Sol understands. He doesn't like it anymore than I do, but he knows I have to take this last step toward completeness. "Go for it!" is his goodbye wish.

"You are truly courageous," Tommy says when I tell him about the impending operation. I protest. "Courageous" is not a word I'd apply to myself. Maybe when I was younger and dumber, although foolhardy is now the way I'd describe my purple heart with an oak leaf cluster.

"You have walked through hell and are about to do it again. That takes courage. I don't know a lot of people who could do it."

I hadn't looked at it that way. To me, it was just doing what I felt had to be done. That's far from being a hero. Heros are daring; I was merely pragmatic.

"It's the way you face up to the fire. You don't flinch. You don't whimper. You just dive in. That's courage, man."

As always, Tommy is immensely encouraging. I'm walking taller. Heroes don't slouch.

Mel has me describe the device in detail and explain where every part goes. He shivers at each detail, but has fun with the pump being located in my scrotum. "You have to be careful when you're making love or, oops, sorry, you must have squeezed my pump! Hand me the Kleenex!"

My son approves of where I'm headed, but has a more practical take on the matter. To wit: if there's a choice of which side of the scrotal pouch the pump is to be installed in, I'd better choose carefully, decide which hand I'd favor as the one to do the pumping because, as a born lefty, he's all-too aware of how trying it is to be on the wrong side of the way most of the world works. Albeit riddled with laughs, this was a serious conversation pursued with love, of which there is no better.

My daughter is thrilled to tears knowing I might soon be able to get out of the box she knows I've been living in since the operation. She kids me about my being able to have sex again—that is, if I'm not too old. A true joy, that girl.

Out of all my other friends and business associates, no one's heard anything about this implant procedure, let alone knows anyone who might know someone who does. A networking dead end, except the Cleveland Clinic winds up scoring points. According to Mel's then partner, it was named one of America's ten best hospitals by *U.S. News & World Report*, and was listed among the best in the country in urology and a dozen other disciplines. Cross off one-story, cinderblock taxpayer.

The question of joining a support group was never a question. I didn't want to come out of the water closet in public. I'd shared enough misery and survived so far, done very well in fact, without the kindness of strangers. Besides, what more could I have learned about incontinence or how to cope? I had a master's degree in the subject. It was too late for patience, hope or more Kegel exercises. Information? Unless it was specifically about the AMS 800 urinary sphincter and how well it worked, I didn't want to hear it. I had all the support I needed from my family and extended family. Like the cowardly lion, what I needed was heart.

I didn't forget to keep Doctor Tom up to date:

March 5, 1996
Dear Tom,

My plumbing repair is scheduled for April 16th. It works out like this: Day 1, a 3-hour physical prep, including a cystoscope; Day 2, the actual procedure; Days 3, 4 and possibly 5, hospital stay, catheterized; Day 5 (or 6, depending) return home, coming back 6 weeks later for Montague to activate the mechanism and ensure that it's in working order. That is, if at any time during the healing, an infection doesn't force him to remove the pump device; or the body, for some reason, rejects it. But that, Montague says, happens in but a small percentage of cases. Since his claimed success rate is 90%, I can only hope the odds are with me this time around. He also says that even with a successful implant, there will be a residual drip or two when sneezing, coughing or sitting on a hard surface too long, requir-

ing only a small pad in one's briefs for the occasional leakage. I'd settle for that. Per Montague's estimate, the freight for this, including hospital, anaesthesia, medication, the works— but excluding travel and expenses— will come to around eighteen thousand. I don't know the insurance ramifications yet, but Dr. M's insurance person will be in touch with me to explain how it works and provide me with a breakdown of the hospital costs. Speaking of hospitals, I find that everytime I mention the Cleveland Clinic, it elicits the kind of awe one usually hears when you mention a place like Johns Hopkins or the Mayo. I'm sure it's no news to you that it's a fine hospital, but it's still encouraging to hear people rave about it. And from the little phone contact I've had with them so far, they sound incredibly efficient. There's even an Omni hotel connected to the hospital, so it'll be convenient for Rose, who's riding shotgun on this trip.

Forgive me, Tom, for going into such detail, but I thought that, as a pioneer, I should share the information with you, so that you, in turn, can share it with other patients you might be recommending this procedure to.

I'll keep you posted.

In a note from Tom, in which he thanks me for keeping him informed of my progress, he concludes with this about Doctor Montague: "Everything I read and hear about him is that he is the Best in the West." A nice uplift from, for my money, the Best in the South.

The Cleveland Clinic lives up to its reputation. One phone call and I am registered, scheduled, instructed, insuranced (sic) and totally impressed. Let's hope they wash their hands as well as they administer.

Time before the trip to Cleveland passes quickly and quietly. I've managed to crawl into an emotional limbo, the heavenly and hellish aspects of my condition beyond my reach. The hermit hibernates, security blanket drawn to his chin, in his fist a nugget of hope that his continence mechanism might yet awaken, aborting the implant mission.

Every day is opening day for me as I tread the boards of my imagination. At least now I know why I don't get the part: I'm too wet. That fact, combined with the thick skin I've acquired, diminishes rejection's power to crush as it once used to. Until the last day, I light candles, genuflect and pray for redemption, hoping that if continence returns, it will do so before I have to get on the plane.

The Cleveland Clinic is big enough to have its own zip code. It isn't so much a hospital as a small city, with many of its buildings connected by a glass-enclosed skyway. Since it is endowed by oil-rich Saudi Arabia, many of its patients are Saudis come to be healed in this state-of-the-art facility, enough so that the hotel's room service menu is printed in Arabic as well as English, and its restaurant features Middle Eastern dishes for dinner.

The story, as told to me by a reliable source—a Cleveland cab driver—is this: years ago, the old Saudi king had a heart problem his country's doctors couldn't fix, so he went to the Clinic and was cured, praise Allah. So grateful was the king, he donated serious oil money to the hospital. Also, since the people in his country have less than ideal life style habits—smoking, fatty and salt-laden diets, insufficient exercise—the king pays for his subjects to visit the Clinic to get their hearts (and no doubt various other organs) repaired, providing a steady flow of patients.

The reception area of the Clinic is a huge mall, several stories high, ringed by balconies and walkways. Hordes of people mill about and wait their turn for admission, a confusing process for the waitees, but ultimately worked out by an unflaggingly-pleasant and efficient cadre.

The efficiency of vitals taken in a room right off the mall so that when you arrive at your eventual medical destination you're at start, not begin, is as awe-inspiring as the hospital's architecture and the Frank Stella hanging on a gallery wall off one of the skyways.

Campus map, assorted papers and newly-issued hospital credit card in hand, I immediately begin to head the wrong way. Were it not for Rose and her sure sense of direction, I'd still be wandering the halls in search of the urology department.

While we're waiting amongst the crowd for one of a roster of urologists, I tell Rose to go back to the hotel since this preoperative checkout is going to take a couple of three hours, and that I can find my way back to the hotel now that I've traversed the route.

"Are you sure?" Rose asks.

"Of course! When I get out of here, I make a right . . . "

"A left."

" . . . to the elevators, then down to the first floor . . . "

"Second floor."

" . . . then I . . . "

"I'll come back to pick you up," Rose says, blowing me a kiss.

After blood, urine, an electrocardiogram and a complete medical history are taken, and I get to choose my favorite anaesthetic for the operation (I opt for a spinal this time around, the memories of recovery from general anaesthesia still too fresh), it is time to meet Doctor Montague.

He is of medium height, impeccably dressed in a well-tailored, dark blue suit, his white beard neatly trimmed; the very model of a department head. Pleasant, yet professionally-distant, Montague quickly allays my fears of being cystoscoped (the memory of having to be put to sleep before they inserted what looked like a broom handle into my penis still haunted me over a dozen years later), explaining that the modern cystoscopic instrument is totally unlike what I remembered.

The procedure isn't painful, but it is disconcertingly unpleasant. To insert the cystoscope, the penis has to be stretched out to create a straight passage for the heavily-KY'd instrument. Once in, both it and the penis then have to be tugged on, twisted and jiggled around in order for the doctor to thoroughly examine the urethral tract. Needless to say, the body is abhoring every second of this trespass.

There is emotional discomfort, too, in that, diaper off, I'm leaking all over the examining table. To the doctor and his nurse, it could have been a gentle spring rain for all the attention they paid to my downpour.

In all fairness, the procedure is over quickly, and the body has to admit it wasn't so bad after all.

"You have a large stricture," Montague says, a problematic edge to his voice.

"Does it pose a problem?" I ask instead of screaming: "Don't tell me I came all the way here to be bumped because of some lousy stricture!"

"It could . . . we'd have to dilate it," he answers, engrossed in my inner topography, obviously weighing the risks versus the rewards.

"You have my permission to dilate, if that counts," I offer.

For the first time, I get a smile, hoping I haven't said something I'll regret down the line.

"Okay, we'll go ahead," he says, mind made up. "Any questions about tomorrow?"

"Do I have a choice as to which side the pump is located in?"

"No. It goes on the left." No debate, but I'm not disappointed since that's the side I had chosen.

"If there are no more questions, I'll see you tomorrow." A

quick handshake, a big smile, and the good doctor is off to keep up with what is obviously a grueling schedule.

Tomorrow's operation doesn't create the same level of anxiety the radical did. It is a relatively quick procedure, doesn't have a life-hanging-in-the-balance quality to it, and it is a finish, it is to be hoped, to this disagreeable episode in our life.

Any residual unease the evening before the operation is erased by the music that pulls us into the hotel's massive lounge as we return from the Clinic. It comes from a jazz duo—piano and standup bass. For over an hour, the two brilliantly explore the standards, finding new roads to wend and higher mountains to climb over old, treasured territory, keeping us exhilarated for hours afterward, tomorrow forgotten in the glow of this serendipitous concert.

"How come you didn't have your radical done here?" asks the amiable anaesthesist as we wait in the hallway for the OR to be ready for us.

"Frankly, I'd never heard of the Clinic until I needed this prosthesis."

"They do great work here," he says with a modest pride, though the implication is that if my radical had indeed, been done here, I might not have had to come back for this implant.

"You mean no patients are left incontinent here?"

"Well, there's a small percentage . . . "

I offer him my hand over the bars of the gurney. "Meet one of the small percentage." Mid-shake, a nurse calls out "Showtime!" and I'm rolled towards the open door.

The operating theater is a giant stage, brilliantly lit, a shadowless movie set of a cutting edge surgical facility, which I'm checking out intently to divert as much attention as I can from the spinal procedure.

"Bend forward from the waist," the anaesthesist gently commands as he lets his fingers do the walking over my lower vertebrae. Once satisfied he's at the right juncture, he swabs the area and lets me know that what's upcoming will be a little uncomfortable. *Everybody knows that when they tell you it's gonna be a little uncomfortable that's a euphemism for godawful. Anyway, was there anything I could do about it? And it's my spine we're talking about for godsakes. Anything could go wrong. Maybe I should have gone with the general anaesthesia.*

"You can lie down now," the anaesthesist is saying.

It's over? A tiny, fleeting bite and a moment of intrusive wiggling is all there was to it? What a waste of good adrenaline!

While I'm prone, a scrim is erected over my chest, separating me from an operation I wasn't about to watch again, especially since it was me under the lights this time. Actually, it doesn't matter, because from the waist down, I don't exist. Were it not for an occasional tug, for all I knew, Doctor Montague and his surgical team could have been in another OR.

Midway through the procedure, I feel myself getting cold, cold enough so that all my upper body muscles are rubbing together to keep warm, so violently, I fear that the vibrations may interfere with the goings on down below. My discomfort doesn't go unnoticed, nor is it unexpected. The anaesthesist explains that the chill is a concomitant of the spinal and the ambient room temperature as he quickly tucks blankets—already heated for this eventuality—all around me. The warmth quickly subdues the shakes, but it's a while before my teeth stop chattering. The last time I felt so chilled was during the Cold War back in the prehistoric era of the mid-fifties, when I had to ride in the open back of a deuce-and-half truck during an alert exercise in the middle of a fierce German winter.

"We're done, Bert," Doctor Montague tells me as he appears from around the screen.

"Everything in place?"

"Everthing in place. I'll see you later."

I think he's smiling under his mask, but I'm not sure, since he moves too quickly to his next assignment.

If I had known recovery from a spinal anaesthetic was such a bore, I would have tried to smuggle in a crossword puzzle.

When my toes, after an aeon of ennui, can discern a pinprick, I'm delivered to my room and my Rose, who fusses over me until I grab one of her hands and kiss it.

"It's over," I tell her, welling up.

She agrees, nodding her head, holding her sobs in with a tissue.

In our joy, we forget the old saw about the fat lady having to sing before the game is actually over.

From my first vitals-taking, I check out my temperature with the nurses, fretting over as small as a one-tenth rise. It's common knowldge that one sign of a rejection is a high fever. Swelling in and around the area is the other indication that everything's not right in implant city. So I'm on alert day and night. It's not that I don't trust Clinic staff, it's because I'm a victim of one of the Percoset painkillers' side effects: agitation. Granted, there is no pain during this three day hospital stint, but I was as wired as if I had downed a ten cup pot of espresso at each of my meals. Speaking of which, the Clinic's food turns out to be the same as at St. Joe's, with identical menus, silverware, dishes. And even with the food on a tray pulled up to your chest, your nose inches from the plates, there's the ultimate similarity: no aroma. My suggestion vis-a-vis Greek diner management still stands.

Petty carping and niggling over hospital food aside (truth is, I had little appetite to begin with), it's the nursing staff at the Clinic that makes the visit bearable, almost pleasant. To a nurse, the staff at the Clinic reflects the unimaginable niceness of all the native Clevelanders we encountered on this trip. Open, caring, professional, unendingly cheerful, funny, smart; they were all of these and more. I am as confident as those who believe there are alien abductions, that Cleveland has developed a secret remedy for good will which, for the sake of the entire world, they should reveal to all of us at the earliest. The nurses have the formula.

"Blood clots look to be the problem," Doctor Matin, one of Montague's assistants says as he palpates my distended bladder. The catheter's out, but the urine refuses to pass, and I know that that spells trouble. Nothing like a shot of adrenaline with your caffeine overload. My mouth is so dry, I can barely ask what has to be done to solve the problem.

Doctor Matin is calm itself.

"Lie down," he says, taking my hands and guiding them into position over the bladder. "Feel the shape." He directs my fingers over the apex. "Here . . . right around here. Push down and away, firmly. Yes, there."

In a burst, urine and blood clots are expelled, instantly relieving the immense pressure and, of course, wetting and staining all the bedclothes. I'd become used to a constant drip, but a torrent, replete with dark red, thick components is too much to let go by without an inner cringe of distress.

Doctor Matin tut-tuts my obvious dismay. "It happens. As long as it's cleared out, that's all that counts."

"Will I be able to go home tomorrow?" I ask.

From the way he's frowning, the answer is no, so I play my last card.

"What if I check out of the hospital today and stay next door in the hotel for another day?"

"As long as you come right back if there are any problems."

"But if everything *is* okay, I can go home the next morning?"

"Just call me before you go and let me know everything is all right. All right?"

I promise the serious, young urology doctor that I will keep him informed.

On a last stroll through the hallways, killing time until I'm granted official release, Doctor Montague joins Rose and me for an au revoir till six weeks from now, adding his best wishes for an uneventful recovery, and reiterating Doctor Matin's directive to call at any time with any questions or problems. His words would have been more of a comfort if we weren't going to be separated by over a thousand miles.

The extra day in the hotel would have been a lot more enjoyable if I could have lolled around in bed until we had to leave for the airport. Instead, I spend half the time trying to placate my bladder, which won't relax until all the debris is flushed out, the other half, dreading the implications of an edgy bladder versus a plane's narrow aisles, and even narrower lavatories.

At the airport, Rose decides that a wheelchair should take me to the gate. When I protest, she says to both me and the wheelchair attendant, "It is too far for you, for him, to walk, and with your, with his, less than rapid pace he'd, we'd, wind up missing the plane, so sit down and shut up, not you. Gate 92, please." Then walks off toward the terminal, with me being pushed behind her.

Thanks to my trusty plastic inner tube and a full dose of Percosets, neither the taxi to the airport, the wheelchair ride to the terminal, the plane trip to Tampa, nor the ride to Treasure Island bother my still tender groin.

As always, it is delicious to be back home, but my pussycats are not sure I am the same person they know. I can almost hear them thinking as they pose, just out of reach, that his voice may be right, but his smell is all wrong. Papa cat should not smell like iodoform and jet fuel. But maybe if he gives us our dinner, we'll forgive him the unsettling odors and welcome him back with lots of leg brushings and purrs. Eager to get back into their good graces, I dutifully dole out their current favorite onto two plates, and out of habit, crouch down to serve them. Wrong move. As I sink down on my haunches, there is a sudden, wrenching pain in my groin, which causes me to drop the plates, the clatter scaring the cats away.

It feels like I've been kicked below the belt, yet I could kick myself for having brought it on. It would have been easy to blame Doctor Montague for not including *Don't Do Deep Knee Bends!* on the no-no list, but how could he have known some patient would hunker down with a bunch of hungry felines like a Papa cat should do?

Happily, the pain doesn't last, but I make a note to, at least until I'm fully healed, feed the cats bending from the waist. They'll have to settle for Papa Butler.

There's nothing like a medical emergency on a Sunday evening to truly spoil a weekend. No matter how good a time was had, it's all forgotten, except for that time-worn knot in your stomach which tightens like it used to when you were a kid, faced with having to go back to school Monday morning.

I had neglected to check my diaper since coming home. When I did, I found it was barely damp when it should have been soaked. And when I stood, I didn't drip. I *had* to drip. I was to be incontinent until the prosthesis was activated. The irony of this is not lost on me. For over a year, I've prayed the dripping would stop, and here I am praying it start again. If I'm not dripping, I realize I could be in serious trouble if whatever is blocking the flow is not cleared. It's "do something" time. Getting catheterized at a local hospital (none of which I was acquainted with) was a less than appealing thought, especially on a Sunday night. I dialed the Clinic's 800 number.

"Cleveland Clinic. How may I help you?"

"I'm calling from Florida . . . and I think I have a medical emergency, and—"

"What department, sir?"

"Urology."

"I'll connect you."

"Urology, Doctor Matin speaking."

Doctor Matin? Doctor Montague's Doctor Matin? I can feel the knot loosening.

"Doctor, this is Bert Gottlieb. I saw you this morning . . . "

"Yes, of course. What seems to be the trouble?"

I tell him, already comforted by his soft voice.

"If we can't clear it up, you'll have to be catheterized," he says, immediately adding, "But I think we can clear it up."

He then proceeds, in his infinitely calm manner, to remind me of the bladder manipulation he taught me when, in the hospital, I had difficulty passing clotted blood, requesting I give the procedure a try, that it should work, and when it did, to let him know, and that if he didn't hear from me in an hour, he'd call me. I was not stranded in St. Petersburg, far from my primary medical source; my doctor had me cradled under his chin. Knot's gone.

Now that I have what I hope is the answer, I tell Rose. She hurriedly takes out rubber sheets and a mountain of towels, preps the bed, and has me lie down and begin my ministrations before I've finished explaining the details.

One good push is all it takes before the sheets and towels are awash with blood clots and urine and my bladder is at peace for the moment, as are the both of us.

As soon as we clean up the place and get the washing machine loaded, I call Doctor Matin to tell him of our success. He sounds as pleased as I am, happy to have been of help, and reminds me to call if anything at all comes up, or if I have any questions about anything, leaving me wondering why I ever worried about the Cleveland Clinic being too far away for comfort.

It takes a few more days for the clotted blood to be fully cleared out, but I've abandoned the bed and the mess created by the bladder-starting maneuver for a cleaner venue: the bathtub. Lay down. Palpate the bladder. Rinse myself and tub off. Done.

The last time I have to go through the routine turns out to be the worst. The mother of all clots is no doubt defending its turf, repelling any chance at relief. Mindful of Doctor Matin's warning not to overdo these bladder squeezes lest the bladder forget how to do them itself, I'm at try three and the bladder is still laboring to void, but getting nowhere, and in spite of the chill of the tub, I'm starting to sweat. Please, let it not be catheter time.

Hands in position, I push down, slowly and firmly. The urge to void is overwhelming. I continue my downward pressure against the unyielding back pressure.

Something—I hope not my bladder, which feels as if it's about to burst—has got to give. It does, in an explosion of huge clots, unlike any I'd seen before, followed by a clear stream of urine. I think the battle is won, the blockade over. Time to heal.

* * *

Chapter 10
Final Admission

Of the six weeks before the next trip to Cleveland, two thirds of them are hellish. When I stand up for more than a few minutes, the pain in my groin forces me to lie down. For a month, I am a bed potato. On my back, the toothache in my crotch is lessened, but never completely gone. More Percosets would no doubt have helped, but they also would (and did) tend to constipate, and the last thing someone whose scrotum has been cut wants to do, is bear down. A dose in the morning and another in the evening were all the drugs I permitted myself. In hindsight, I should have known it would be a rough recovery by the generous quantity of painkillers that had been prescribed.

After a few days of nothing but bed, Rose can see I am becoming a basketcase and should be, pain or no, up and about a bit more.

"Here's the deal," she says. "I'm gonna shop and you're gonna cook. How's that sound?"

"You know I can't stand up for too long," I whine.

"You'll work it out." No mercy.

I do work it out: it's peel and cut an onion, run to the living room clutching my crotch, plunk down on the couch until the awful ache abates, then back to the range to heat oil in the pan and start the onions sauteeing, the couch-to-kitchen-to couch routine continuing until dinner is ready.

Cleaning up afterwards is as much of a Marx Brothers romp as is the cooking. My imitation of Groucho's crouch as I run between rooms is an award-winning performance by any standard.

The thought that the implant might be rejected is never far from the surface, even though my temperature is normal and there is no evidence of swelling or tenderness anywhere in the vicinity of the implant. Like the persistent, throbbing, knee-buckling pain (except when the Percosets are at work), the thought never goes away. Until a month to the day.

Getting out of bed that day, I realize there is no pain as I stand up. It is so hard to believe, I have to take a few tentative steps to assure myself that I'm not still asleep. Convinced, I walk decidedly into the kitchen, where Rose is getting ready to boil some water.

"What are you doing up?" she scolds.

I hold a finger to my lips and whisper, "Don't say a word, but I think the pain is gone."

"Are you sure?" she whispers back.

"I'm sure," I answer, pirouetting round the kitchen.

"Great. Make me a cup of tea then."

"Poof. You're a cup of tea."

While we're laughing and hugging, I make a note to mark this milestone day on our perpetual calendar.

Before I am to return to Cleveland for the start-up procedure, Doctor Montague dictated this informative courtesy letter, which Tom thoughtfully faxed me a copy of.

Dear Dr. Mawn:

On April 9, 1996, I implanted an artificial urinary sphincter in Mr. Gottlieb for treatment of urinary incontinence status post radical retropublic prostatectomy. Preoperative cystoscopy revealed a wide caliber stricture at the bladder neck. During the operation we dilated this to 20 French with filiforms and follow-

ers and we placed a 16 French Foley.

Mr. Gottlieb did well postoperatively. The catheter was removed on the third postoperative day, and following catheter removal, there was some bleeding and some clot retention. We did not have to reinstrument him as he started voiding, but with difficulty. We kept him in the hospital an extra length of time until he was voiding satisfactorily.

He was discharged on April 13, 1996. The device is deactivated. Mr. Gottlieb is returning in approximately six weeks for a postoperative visit and for activation of the prosthesis and instruction in its use.

Thank you for the opportunity of sharing in his care.

May 29, 1996 is another day that has to go down in the books. It's Wednesday in Cleveland and I'm at the Clinic in one of the examining rooms. Doctors Montague and Matin are pondering my left testicle, mumbling out of earshot. Doctor Montague reaches into my scrotum and tugs at something a few times, eliciting a noisy gasp from me. But he is not to be deterred. He apologizes for causing me the discomfort, explaining that somehow the pump is upside down—not a problem with kink-proof tubing—and will just have to be dealt with from a different perspective.

"You mean it's already activated?"

"Yes," Montague says, adding, "Now we have to check it out, make sure it works, and that you can work it." He pours me a giant tumbler of water. "Drink this, relax, read a book. I'll be back in about 20 minutes and we'll test it out."

Twenty minutes. It's taken over two years to get within shouting distance of the finish line. I can wait. I can stare out the window at the chilly Spring landscape and know that, in no time, I'll be inhaling that promising end-of-winter air, a free man, no more a prisoner of my damaged body. From now on, I could come and go as I pleased without thinking about whether I needed a change of diaper. No more would my penis always look as if it had stayed in a swimming pool too long. I can wait. Who can't wait for dessert?

By the time twenty minutes have passed, I find I can't wait. My bladder is p-mailing me distress messages. Doctor Montague arrives in time to show me the actual device, explain how it has rotated, and how to go about activating it.

Standing in front of a stainless steel sink cum urinal, I fumble for the pump, trying to get my thumb and index finger oriented to its topography, all the while staring at the prosthesis the doctor is holding in his palm, a tiny, plastic jewel of a mechanism. When I think I've located the right spot, I give the pump a tentative squeeze, followed by, at the urging of Montague, a more sure one. For a moment, nothing happens, then bingo, it is working; I am urinating. I am back. It is over. Out of the corner of my eye, I can see Doctor Montague quietly smiling as he makes his notes. As commonplace a procedure as this no doubt is for him, I'm confident he's pleased at every successful implant, mine being no exception. I cannot, of course, stop grinning as I thank him for all he's done, and bid him goodbye.

The grin fades a bit thirty-thousand feet or so over the Florida panhandle when I boldly go where everyone's gone before: the plane's lavatory.

It's enough of a trick to pee in a plane under normal circumstances; try, in a cramped, bouncing space, to find a small, unfamiliar, wiggly object in your scrotum and get it to hold still long enough to be squeezed, being careful not to squeeze the wrong part of the pump (which would keep the collar open), or the spermatic cords (which would feel like you've been kicked below the belt).

Success comes, but not without a price: I forget to wait the extra minute until the sphincter collar is fully closed, and wind up spotting my slacks. Slinking back to my seat, I swear never to forget the added time the device needs to close off the urethra.

By the time we get to Tampa, my pants are dry and my grin is back.

It is a sunny Tampa Bay day as the plane touches down, made even sunnier by my family being at the airport to greet me and haul my happy ass home.

The evening is such a blur of stale pump jokes, exotic cold beer and familial warmth, I can recall only one conversation.

I had put off buying another package of diapers, rationing what I had on hand till this day, making sure there were a couple left, just in case. However, what I needed now was an absorbent pad, an area of purchase I knew nothing about.

I beckon to the family's acknowledged shopping maven, my daughter, and explain my need. In a nanosecond she retrieves the answer from her huge mental database, and allows as since she is going out, she'll pick me up a package on her way home.

It turns out to be Always Ultra-Thin Maxi Pads with Wings. When I ask why they need wings, Lori explains that the wings hold the pads in place in one's briefs. Who was I to argue with perhaps one of America's premier shoppers.

She is right, of course; Always always work, as a hack copy-writer might headline an ad. Not that I haven't looked into other brands. After standing in front of my supermarket's sanitary napkin display for much too long, I still couldn't figure out which of the myriad pad offerings would do. The varieties of brands, absorptive qualities, thicknesses, curves, shapes and the non-universal language from product to product, had me utterly confused, so I chose to stick with the brand I had started with. Why I ever thought I'd outshop a pro is beyond me. It would be nice, though, if the Always package were blue, rather than pink.

It isn't until after a shower the next morning that I begin to feel like a whole person again. Save for the quirky little maneuver I have to go through to urinate, it is a heady feeling to feel like the same man I was before. No more a prisoner locked in solitary, I can walk in the sunlight, free of the velcro shackles.

I'm neither a nudist, nor have I flasher tendencies, but it is a thrill to be able to walk around without anything on. Not to be able to perform the simple, most natural act of walking naked from a shower to a bedroom a few feet away, can only be described as living in a cell without walls; it is days before I can allow myself to appreciate their disappearance. It takes time to forget what was and accept what is. There's also a wariness I suspect comes with age, that allows us to defer our pleasures until we're sure a celebration is in order. And so I tiptoe into freedom, feeling my way until I'm confident enough to appreciate the fact that I'm out of captivity for good.

A week after I'm home, Rose asks me if, now that I'm dry, it would be okay to have sex. I can't remember what I answered, nor if I answered at all, but as happens in second-rate novels, before we knew it we were pulling at each other's clothes, two teenagers who couldn't get to it quickly enough.

Afterwards, pleased and amused at our wham-bam-thank-you, ma'am performance, we allow as how having to wait two years to sate our hunger for each other had starved us into swallowing our food almost without tasting it.

We promise ourselves, between giggles and hugs, that we'll take our time next time.

I sleep deeply, dream-free and, not since the night before the first operation, in the raw. The nightmare is over. I think I can hear the fat lady singing.

While the pump works exceedingly well, by the nature of its location, it calls attention to itself.

As the reserve of liquid begins to flow back to the collar,

swelling it to lock off the urethral flow, the local nerves, stimulated unnaturally, seem to be receiving mixed signals as the collar tightens. There's the relief of having voided, and disconcertingly, on its heels, the urge to void. Until the feelings pass, it's like facing a stoplight that's registering red and green at the same time. You don't know, as the expression goes, and seems to fit as never before, "whether to piss or wind your watch."

Also, come a chilly morning, when one's scrotum has most naturally tightened up and shrunk as far into the body cavity as it can in order to maintain the body's preferred testicular temperature, try and find the "go" part of the pump without squeezing a hunk of spermatic cord.

Stress incontinence continues as promised and predicted. A heavy sneeze or cough, or sitting on a hard surface for too long a time (however long *that* is I haven't figured out yet), will definitely push a few drops past the collar. Mind, I'm not complaining. I'm *this* close to whole again, and that's good enough, all things considered.

Early in June, Doctor Montague sends me a copy of his followup letter to Doctor Tom.

Dear Dr. Mawn:

On May 29, 1996, Bert Gottlieb returned for a postoperative visit. He was voiding well and incontinent as before the surgery. Examination revealed that his incisions were well healed and urinalysis was negative. The pump is in the left hemiscrotum, but has migrated to the upper portion of the scrotum and is upside down. Fortunately, with kink-proof tubing, this does not present a problem in the functioning of the device.

Once again, thank you for the opportunity of sharing in his care. If his continence is satisfactory, I will not need to see him again. I told him to give me a call if he is having any problems.

It's a spring-like Florida day this September ninth, and my walk must reflect it as I stride into Doctor Tom's examining room. I'm anxious for my PSA test results (the last one was seven months ago), and to show him the new, straighter, taller, happier me.

"You look great," he says as we shake hands. His smile says it even more positively.

It is obvious how pleased he is that I have survived both as a patient and, after a relationship of over two years, as a friend. We have, in our dealings with each other gone beyond doctor-patient linkage to something even more intimate: kinship. We may be related solely by prostate, but that doesn't make the fondness any less.

Friendship aside, I am told to drop my Dockers for the ever-popular DRE. But first, anxious to check out the device, Tom fingers my scrotum, tracing the outline of the pump mechanism, seeing how it sits in the sac, making mental doctor notes.

"By the way, Bert, your PSA is less than 0.2."

Imagine, I forgot to ask. Even though the PSA result was the first thing on my mind, how quickly it got overlooked amidst the ca-maraderie and good cheer of the visit. For a moment I questioned whether I was being overconfident, perhaps even blase, but quickly reject the notion, because there's no such thing as overconfidence when it comes to prostate cancer—not until I (and every patient like me) don't have to see a doctor for a checkup anymore. With life back, the darker possibilities have been banished to a dim corner. They are allowed to sneak out into the light every so often, but once the visit is over, they're again consigned to the shadows .

I feel as good leaving Tom's office today as I did the first time I left, the time he told me my BPH symptoms didn't warrant any concern, the time a lifetime ago, when I wanted to light up a smuggled Monte Cristo and celebrate my good fortune, .

Daybook Entry, 9/4/96

Patient: BG
PSA: O.2 Ng/Ml
DRE: Felt no induration of the prostatic fossa.
Reason for visit: 27 month post-op checkup.
Management: Return in 6 months, with PSA prior to visit.
Post Visit Thoughts & Observations: Bert is doing exceedingly
well. He is, once again, a complete man, and I am happy for him.
It's been a hard road to travel, but he's survived the journey with
dignity, patience and, amazingly, good humor. Due to the vagar-
ies of cancer cells, he will always be my patient and, in spite of
whatever direction they might decide to go in, my friend as well.

Each post-op visit that registers negative for prostate antigen activity
is cause to celebrate. This time we go a little overboard. After a
couple of three glasses of bubbly, toasts are still forthcoming.

     "Here's to survival," I cheer, finishing my glass in a gulp.

     "To Doctor Tom," Rose counters, emptying her glass, too.

     "To May twenty-seventh, ninteen ninety-four."

     "Huh?"

     "That's the day of the operation—the day the cancer died."

     "I'll drink to that, if I had anything to drink."

     I crack open another bottle, and after a symbolically dripless
pour, raise my glass. "To May twenty-ninth, nineteen ninety-six."

     "May twenty-ninth?"

     "The day the pump went into operation."

     "Oh, yeah. I'll drink to that."

     "To Ziggy, may he— "

     "Who's Ziggy?"

     "My conscience. It's a long story. Cheers."

     "Cheers, my love."

Chapter 11
Acceptance Speech

Fellow members, spouses, visitors: as I stand before you, having had a couple of years to reflect on everything that's transpired, permit me to sum up my experiences, underscore some of the lessons to be taken away, and of course, talk much too much.

First, I want to thank the Club for this honor it has bestowed upon me: the Order of the Golden Walnut, acknowledgment of my survival of the "biggie," with lapel button, tie tack, cufflinks, bumper stickers and T-shirts available for purchase in the lounge.

My decision to undergo a radical was not easy; it never is, as I needn't tell any of the club members. Nor would the choice of any other treatment have been any easier. Everything in our struggle against prostate cancer is hard; decisions hardest— with fear being the most palpable emotion and, at times, the most mind-numbing.

Speaking of emotions, it's a wonder humor isn't considered one. Don't we laugh until we cry, laugh our hearts out, laugh ourselves to death? Humor is a defense against spurious emotions, and laughter is good medicine in spite of the fact that you can't get a prescription for it. If you can laugh at the fates, maybe you can deflect their attention and alter their calendar of events; if you don't succeed, it wouldn't be for not trying. When we exercise our sense of humor, we not only embolden our spirits to fly above the fearful events that are taking place within us, according to growing research, there's a link between laughter and strengthened immune systems, recovery from illness, improved muscle tone, lowered blood pressure, raised pain thresholds and reduced stress. With all that going for it, it shouldn't be long before a book entitled *Laughing Yourself to Wellness* hits the non-fiction charts.

Even urologists laugh at themselves.

Marcel Proust's younger brother, Robert, a surgeon, was so well-known for doing prostatectomies, that in his circle, they were called "proustatectomies." Not exactly a thigh-slapper, but perhaps it was the doctors' way of shrugging off the depressing emotions that surrounded what was then (and still is) a bloody awful procedure, the "if we didn't laugh, we'd cry" syndrome.

Urologists, naturally, are the butt of many jokes. We've all heard the line, "Never accept a drink from a urologist." Or "Urologists are the only doctors who carefully wash their hands before they pee." And who hasn't encountered the by now stale, but enduring, "the time to get nervous when undergoing a digital rectal examination, is when the doctor puts both his hands on your shoulder."

In spite of the sexist (there are women urologists) and homophobic aspects of this joke, as with all good humor, it's the unexpected turning of logic on its head which prompts the laugh and permits the release of bedeviling emotions, not the least of which is fear, particularly that of invasion, even if it's only by a finger. No matter how many times a man has to submit to a DRE, it is a disconcerting experience having someone poke around inside his rectum. The real joke, as we all know too well, is where the prostate is located.

Unfortunately, prostate cancer is not funny and must be taken seriously. After age 50 (or earlier if there's a known genetic disposition to prostate difficulties) a man's prostate should be checked out yearly by a doctor's educated digit and a PSA test taken because, in most instances, the results can indicate the presence of cancer as early as five years before any other means. And since all treatments can work better at a low PSA, the earlier any indications of trouble in Prostate City, the better the chances for survival. A man's PSA number should be as well-known to him as his phone number. It's not enough for a man's doctor to stay in touch with his prostate, it's the man's duty as well. If I were the father of the bride in a remake of *The Graduate*, the best advice I could give to the hapless Dustin Hoffman wouldn't be "plastic," it would be "PSA."

Looking back, after all that's transpired, I still feel I made the right decision to undergo a radical prostatectomy. Even after five years of reading, writing, thinking about and living with prostate cancer and its consequences, I would take the same path I took at the beginning of my trip and, needless to say, with the same doctor.

I received the best care, consideration and attention a modern medical practitioner could provide. There wasn't a moment when I felt under-cared for or, worse yet, under-communicated to. Granted, I studied the subject on my own, but every question I asked my doctor always received an answer. There were never any mysteries. If I never picked up a book or talked to another person, I am confident Doctor Tom would still have brought all the skill and dedication he could muster to the task.

Why then, with all that trust, was there such intense study of the subject on my part? With the stakes being so high, I would have been a fool not to have cut the cards, though nothing I learned before, during or after my radical was at variance with anything my urologist ever said. But in fairness to all parties—urologists and patients—how much time, from initial discovery to over and done with, do the parties actually spend together? If I add up my actual face time with Tom—from the inception up to the operation—we're talking three, possibly four hours total, broken mostly into quarter hour segments.

Not enough class time to make an educated decision. Yet how much information can a doctor be expected to impart, especially in such brief spurts, and with stressed emotions fighting for attention? It's a wonder anything of value gets through to a patient under those conditions.

Consider the physician who has great instincts, ethics and experience, but is a lousy communicator. Notwithstanding this physician's sincerity, his medical jargon is worthless if you're not quite sure of what he's talking about. Facts are only valuable if you understand them. Basing a decision on fear, denial, depression, mourning or any other emotions, should be a scarier thought than that of having prostate cancer. With the facts in hand, you're empowered to guide your own destiny. With knowledge, you can make the right-for-you decisions, none of which you'll have reason to regret, no matter what the outcome. Death would, without a doubt, be easier than having to kick yourself in the ass every day of your life for gross stupidity.

According to one prostate cancer guide, I missed experiencing only one of the emotions a freshly-minted prostate cancer victim is expected to encounter: anger. It just wasn't in me to stand on a mountain top, fists raised, yelling, "Why me, damnit?," when I already knew the answer was "Why not?" Adenocarcinoma is a random pathological process that bears no malice; it just does its mutated thing until stopped, or until it kills the host. No one points a finger and says, "Him!"

If someone kicks a man in the crotch, there's every reason to scream foul, but a group of out of control tissues, caused by all the obvious suspects—genetics, the environment, personal life styles, and who knows how many other not so apparent factors—doesn't seem to be much of a reason for anger. Prostate cancer is a vulgar disease, a reflection of the fact that, unfortunately, shit happens.

Dependent on a man's PSA numbers and all the other variables that go into his decision-making, he may or may not walk in my clinical footsteps, but he's sure to cross over some of the emotional paths I took, and will almost certainly find a couple of side roads of his own.

In 1999, it is estimated that 179,300 men will be diagnosed with prostate cancer, and that one of six men will be diagnosed with the disease in their lifetime. (In 1996, the number was 300,000, but the latest statistics show that the incidence of newly-diagnosed prostate cancer is decreasing.) Even so, 37,000 men will die from (not just with) adenocarcinoma. Which makes prostate cancer the number one malignant tumor (excluding skin cancers) afflicting men, and their number two killer.

To that army of 179,300 new recruits (and I'm sure I speak for all Club members), you have our best wishes and our admonition to read and learn all you can about this ugly, albeit most important subject.

Prostate cancer knowledge is readily available, but it's a small shelf of books. Breasts garner the most attention, the most books, and also the most research dollars—close to five times as many as for prostate cancer. Yet I haven't run into a man (including men in their twenties) who didn't want to learn more about this disquieting subject. Women, too, in my experience, seem to be fascinated with our enigmatic gland, aware that they have to stay on top of the issue in the event their partners don't, won't or can't think about it. Let's face it, when detected, prostate cancer winds up being as much a woman's disease as a man's. It may not affect her body, but it attacks her life just as inexorably. To whatever other wifely chores she has to address, we can add caregiver, head of household, therapist, patient advocate, and medical researcher, to name but a few of the new responsibilities facing her.

There is no dirth of newspaper articles about prostate cancer. Problem is, they can be confusing and sometimes contradictory. Take these two headlines: *Exploring the full healing spectrum* and *Beware of alternative therapies.* Same day, same paper, same page. Then there's this trio of headlines that surfaced in '96: *Prostate removal improves chances of survival; Prostate Cancer: Radiation as good as surgery; and Further treatment after "curative" radical prostatectomy often required.* Contradictory? Confusing? Yes. And yes. Which is why, after you think you've learned all you need to know about prostate cancer, question everything you've learned. Network with friends, relatives, acquaintances, anyone and everyone who might have more than a nodding acquaintance with the disease. Go on-line and enter a prostate cancer chat room. Surf the web for additional up-to-date information. Do everything you can to ensure that whatever choices you decide upon, they're based on solid knowledge and close-to-rational decisions, not on the smoke of emotions or any of the other roadblocks to reason. If you some-day want to stand in front of us accepting your golden walnut, rather than having your loved ones standing over you clutching soggy tissues, you'll stay prostate smart.

We all know the famous members of our club: Bob Dole, Norman Schwartzkopf, Arnie Palmer, et al; they are held up as exemplars of prostate cancer survival by the media when it's a dull news day and they've run out of diseases du jour. It might do more good to mention the famous non-members—men like Telly Savalas, Bobby Riggs, Bill Bixby, Francois Mitterand, Don Ameche, Frank Zappa, even the Ayatollah Khomeini. But dying from prostate cancer is somehow considered old news; only surviving seems to merit any ink.

Imagine reading about a woman of celebrity losing a breast cancer battle due to inattention, neglect or some other inexcusable reason. I can't. Nor have I. Nor, hopefully, will I ever, because most of the reasonably-aware female world has gone on breast cancer alert, ready to detect its presence as early as possible.

If I can leave you with but two thoughts, they are: the early PSA catches the cancerous worm; and the primary entry requirement into the club is that you be alive.

Obviously, I share the dais tonight with my doctor and my friend, but before I turn it over to him, I'd like to share this note from my old companion with you. It reads:

Dear Bert,   Sorry I had to run off.   Couldn't face the fact that my guilt trips had no effect in Tampa or St. Petersburg. Am sharing a house in the Hollywood hills with my old friend, Carl Jung. We argue a lot, but we both agree that prostate cancer is a pain.

Live long.

Ziggy.

Common wisdom has it that one should begin a speech with a joke, a little something to warm up one's audience. But unlike Bert, who can somehow manufacture a smile from our grim subject, I can't.

In my practice, I see the unfunny impact of prostate cancer on the all-too many good men who come to me for treatment, and it always eats at me, so that little by little, over the years, it has gnawed away at my funny bone, till—at least on this subject—there's nothing left to laugh about. Even my smiles are rationed, brought out only for successful outcomes and continuing low PSA scores.

There is, though, something mildly amusing in the fact that PSA testing—the single most important factor in revolutionizing prostate cancer management that has occurred in the last fifteen years—had its first clinical application as a forensic tool in cases of alleged rape. The reason: PSA concentration levels in semen are nearly one hundred times that found in blood or serum.

The uncanny specificity of serum PSA to detect prostate (and only prostate) disease provided a new paradigm for urologists and oncologists in the management of both benign and malignant prostate problems—not to mention new life to thousands of men.

Unfortunately, in recent years, a PSA controversy has developed, not in the use of the PSA test to follow the progression of prostate disease; the debate is over whether the test should be used for prostate cancer "screening"—mass testing of a given population for the disease, in an effort to diagnose the incidence of disease, regardless of the presence or absence of any signs or symptoms.

The dilemma is this: on the one horn, mass screening can and will save lives by early detection of "curable" prostate cancers; on the other, it will impact on the lives of those who have been detected with it, as well as require the expenditure of significant quantities of health care resources, both public and private.

With health care spending in the United States hovering around the $1 trillion mark, there is no question that health-care priorities must be established, that complex and oftimes confusing choices have to be made, and that, in the mix, ethical medical questions have also to be included in the considerations.

But how to choose, how to set priorities, how to be fair.

Is medical insurance there to cure (as but an example) infertility and remove birthmarks? Or should it be reserved for only serious illnesses and disabilities?

To the couple who can't conceive, or the person with a disfiguring facial wen, their need for care is as serious as that of someone who needs a hip replacement.

Solomon himself would be daunted by the array of medical treatments available (and asked for) today. Imagine having to choose and prioritize between heart transplants, penile implants, cataract removals, cleft palate repairs, breast reconstructions, AIDs drug regimes, or Prozac prescriptions for an unknown length of time, to name but a few of the treatment possibilities.

But if Solomon's eyes were growing dim, I somehow think his judgments would be swift, with cataract removal high on his medical priorities list.

That said, permit me to mention a few criteria to be met if mass PSA screening is to be justified.

Is prostate cancer a disease that poses a major health threat?

Since prostate cancer is the number one cancer affecting men, and the number two cancer killer of men, there can be no debate here.

Is the PSA test sensitive enough to detect prostate cancer in its early stages?

There is sufficient data to demonstrate that if the PSA result is less than 10 Ng/Ml, there's a fifty percent chance that the tumor will be confined to the prostate, and as such, potentially curable. (At Johns Hopkins, they have defined curability as organ-confined with any grade of cancer, or specimen-confined with a Gleason sum of less or equal to 6. Under this definition, 74% of their patients were curable.[1] Of course, prostate cancer is normally asymptomatic at this stage, and without an early warning marker such as the PSA test provides, there's no sure way to tell where a man's prostate stands.

Are there any studies that show prostate cancer screening reduces the death rate from prostate cancer?

Yes. In a large Canadian trial study, population-based screening for prostate cancer has been proven to decrease the disease-specific mortality rate.[2] The report compared disease stages in patients who were screened and those who were not. The study showed that the screened cases had a lower perecentage of advanced disease, which strongly implied that with screening, the death rate will ultimately decrease.[3,4,5]

Is the PSA test relatively inexpensive in order for screening to become a practical consideration?

As of this writing, in the Southeastern United States, the cost ranges from fifty to seventy dollars per PSA test. However, the "wholesale" price which governments and medical insurance companies would no doubt bargain for, could bring the price down to (an educated guess) as low as fifteen dollars per test. If we include the cost of an office visit, at which time a DRE would be performed, the total cost of a prostate cancer screening could be less than that of a breast cancer mammography screening test.

Do PSA screened patients actually benefit from the results?

If a PSA test reveals prostate cancer that is potentially curable, the answer has to be a resounding yes. Yet not all patients with diagnosed adenocarcinoma need to have treatment. Urologists are well-aware, based on a wealth of transurethral resection pathology reports, that there is a group of patients that have but a microscopic focus of prostate cancer and, that in most such cases, that small foci of prostate carcinoma does not represent a true clinical and possibly lethal disease, and that these men can (and do) lead normal life spans without any further treatment. It is estimated that from seven to ten percent of PSA-screened men will fall into this category.

At the other end of the spectrum, a percentage of men will have been discovered to have very high grade, aggressive cancer, for which no cure is likely by any treatment method.

In the case of older and younger men who have serious concurrent problems such as cardiopulmonary or vascular disease, it is mostly axiomatic that they will not live long enough to die from prostate cancer, rendering any additional measures unnecessary.

In my experience, the benefit derives from knowing either that the cancer is curable, or that it is microscopic in size and not potentially lethal, or that some other disease will take you down before prostate cancer does. There is even some benefit in knowing that one's cancer is incurable and irrevocably fatal if it can help lead to a settling of one's life accounts with closure for all concerned. Any measure that can help soften the landing and dignify the finish has to be considered a plus.

Can we say then, that the benefits of screening warrant the cost?

From the thousands of men who will survive prostate cancer thanks to early diagnosis, and from the other thousands who will be able to breathe a sigh of relief from prostate cancer worries, you will get no argument.

Unfortunately, the carefully planned, statistically sound, randomized studies that would, it was hoped, provide us with definitive answers, are still in the early stages and not yet mature enough to conclusively prove or disprove the efficacy of screening, although some of the most recent data indicate the incidence (or rate) of prostate cancer diagnosis has peaked and finally leveled, and other just published statistics are beginning to show that early diagnosis has, indeed, led to early treatment, with, as a result, the death rate having leveled as well.

So where does the medical community currently stand vis a vis prostate cancer screening?

The spectrum of conclusions and recommendations is wide, ranging from that of the U.S. Preventative Services Task Force, whose position is that prostate cancer screening should not be done at all— to that of the American Urologic Society, which has recommended that digital rectal examinations and PSA determinations be performed annually solely on men over age fifty, and starting at age forty-five in men who are at high risk, i.e., blacks and men with first degree relatives who have had prostate cancer.

The American College of Physicians and the American Cancer Society recommend that each patient first be counseled, and also be willing to undergo biopsy and treatment should prostate cancer be diagnosed as a result of the PSA screening.

Some middle ground has already been met: limiting screening to men between the ages of 50 and 70, and men in the high risk groups, excluding men who would probably not live more than ten years, and would not really benefit from treatment.

Even the American Urologic Association is modifying its recommendations to address this factor. Their rationale is that if any benefit is to occur, it will be in the group most likely to die from prostate cancer if something is not done.

From the "big picture" point of view, screening limitations appear reasonable enough. However, they fail to address the men who don't fit the proscribed profiles, thousands of whom may needlessly face a death sentence as a result of a too late diagnosis.

Limitations of this kind also imply that somehow, physicians will be given divine knowledge as to which side of the picture an individual will arrive at. The light of statistical, cost-benefit reasoning pales when a doctor is faced with a man's life about to ebb from a cancer that could have been detected at an early-enough stage to be cured. And while the cure is, admittedly, not inexpensive, it is far less costly in the long run if the dollars that will be spent on long term terminal care are added up. Or to shorthand it: we can pay now, or we can pay more later. End of speech.

Thank you for your forebearance, and my apologies for not providing lots of laughs, but if I've at least provided something to think about, I deserve that drink I'm going to have with Bert as soon as I step down from the dais. Good night and good health.

* * *

Chapter Footnotes

1 Carter, H.B., Epstein, J.I., Caan, D.W., et al, *Recommended Prostate-Specific Antigen Testing Intervals for the Detection of Curable Prostate Cancer.* JAMA, 1997; 277: 1456-1460.

2 Mitka, M., *Mixed Response to New PSA Screening Study.* JAMA, 1998; 280 8-9.

3 Catalona, W.J., Smith, D.S., Ratliff, T.L., Basler, J.W., *Detection of Organ-Confined Prostate Cancer Increased Through Prostate Specific Antigen Based Screening.* JAMA, 1998; 270; 948-954.

4 Catalona, W.J., *Screening for Prostate Cancer.* New England Journal of Medicine, 1996; 334; 666-667.

5 Moul, J.W., T*reatment Options for Prostate Cancer, Part 1: Stage Grade, PSA, and Changes in the 1990s.* AN Journal of Managed Care, 1998; 4; 1031-1034.

Chapter 12
Epilogue

October 21, 1997 was a perfect, West Central Florida day: low seventies and dry—the natives' Spring, so to speak, payback for the crushing heat and humidity of the long summer, which clammy grip only just now was beginning to loosen. The air was as clear as polished crystal, so delicate and crisp, it seemed as if it would shatter if one blinked too hard.

It is an upbeat day in more ways than one. Save for tidying up, the book that Tom and I have written (this book) is almost completed, awaiting but the ministrations of an understanding and forgiving editor. Also, I'm on my way into Tampa for my every six month PSA cum DRE—by now a ho-hum event—and am looking forward to seeing Doctor Tom. To top if off, I'm days away from becoming a grandfather for the first time, and am as excited as the expectant mother, a wonder, since I'd always thought I lacked grandparental genes.

The day couldn't have been sunnier.

In spite of our busy schedules and the distance between us, Tom and I are in constant touch. We overnight mail, fax and e-mail notes and comments, jabber on the phone. What we don't get to do is see each other face to face too often, so an office visit is something we both look forward to. It's a chance to schmooze a bit, catch up on things other than the book (though I was anxious this day to tell him about an exciting conversation I'd had with a literary agent), all the while perfunctorily going through the post prostate drill.

"No induration of the prostatic fossa?" I ask, as Tom strips off his glove and hands me a box of tissues.

"You're beginning to sound like a urologist."

"Anytime you need a hand, doctor, or should I say a finger."

While we're laughing, and as Tom makes a note that there is, indeed, no induration of the prostatic fossa, I remember to ask about my PSA number.

"It was zero point three . . . but come on into my office and we'll talk," Tom answers.

Zero point three. A click over my last test result. A lousy tenth of a percent higher. What's the big deal? Why can't we talk about it here? I'm not going to like this conversation.

In his office, Tom makes it a point to sit next to me on one of the visitor's chairs instead of behind his desk.

Now, I'm positive I'm not going to like what I'm about to hear.

"Only a few years ago," Tom explains, "the allowable PSA could go as high as zero point five—recall some of your early post-radical PSA scores. But since that time the test has become more refined and sensitive, and the numbers have to register no more than zero point two. Higher than that and we have to consider a possible recurrence."

I could feel the color washing out of my face. It wasn't the thought of dying that made me pale, it was envisioning more precious time out of my life undergoing batteries of tests and who-knows-how-many treatments to rid my body of any prostate cancer leftovers.

I saw days of discomfort and weeks, maybe months, of worry ahead. I felt like retching.

My reaction was obviously apparent, and no doubt expected.

"Are you all right?" Tom asks, trying to keep a bright face, but not succeeding. He looks as bad as I feel.

I shake my head yes, albeit begrudgingly. What can you say when the balloon turns out to be full of hot air and suddenly collapses all around you?

"Are you scared?" Tom asks, squeezing my forearm.

"No, not scared," I answer, once I can get my mouth working again. "Concerned is more like it."

"Look, Bert, it could be a lab variation or a biological fluctuation—"

"How often do those occur?" A hint of testiness has crept into my voice, a sharp edge of cynicism.

"Often enough," Tom answers, ignoring my little outburst, and proceeds to tell me about a colleague whose recent PSA registered normal, even though the DRE didn't, but that a subsequent PSA test agreed with Tom's finger's finding. A follow-up sonogram-biopsy concurred: he did have prostate cancer.

The story did little to encourage me. I felt I had crapped out again.

"What if it's not a variation or fluctuation? What do we do then?" I can't understand how my voice has become so calm when there's such screaming inside my head.

Tom strokes my arm and explains that there's a new diagnostic tool that can identify the exact location of prostate cancer cells specifically, and that with radiation and hormone therapy, if necessary, it can be treated effectively. But before we come to that, he wants another blood test done before I leave the building.

I didn't want to hear what Tom said. I already had a good idea of what the answer would be. It was as if I were hearing I had prostate cancer for the first time. All emotional systems went on line: the back of my thighs started to itch in synch with the bum news; the headache was foreshadowing its entrance by racking up the balls with which it would play pool in my head for a couple of hours; and Izzy was not going to be able to help, being holed up somewhere in Benedict Canyon. I could have cried from disappointment.

" . . . so right after you leave here, get another blood test.

Okay?" Tom's voice swims into my consciousness.

Numbly, I agree, already thinking about how I'm going to break this to Rose.

"Tom, I think . . . I think I'm not going to tell Rose just yet. Let's wait until the results of the next PSA. If it's just a lab deviation, no need to say anything. If it's a recurrence, I can always tell her then."

"No, Bert." Tom is adamant. "You can't lie about this. You've shared everything with her so far. Don't cut her out now. I'll call her if you want."

Tom is right. I can't spare her from this. She'd never forgive me. I'd never forgive me. "I'll tell her."

Daybook Entry, 10/21/97

Patient: *Bert Gottlieb*
PSA: *0.3 Ng/Ml*
DRE: *No induration of prostatic fossa.*
Elevated PSA presents as either possible recurrence or lab variation. If followup PSA remains constant, confirming as recurrence, pinpointing the exact location of the recurrence will be the next course of action.
Followup: *Return in 2 weeks, PSA ASAP prior to visit.*
Post Visit Thoughts & Observations: *I am encouraged by a new, cutting edge prostate cancer detection tool. Since the PSA test is positive proof of recurrence, but doesn't reveal where the recurrent site is, and is often undetectable by MRI or CT scans, this new locating agent (dubbed Prostascint) will help speed up treatment decisions. This is an important advance, since the sooner recurrent cancer is treated, the better the results. The detection agent is made up of antibodies, created to zero in on prostate cancer cells specifically, each molecule of which is identified by a radioactive marker. A*

*gamma camera can then scan the patient and pinpoint wher-
ever the cancer has taken hold, ensuring more accurate treatment decisions.*

    *There is no way to cushion the dismaying news of a pos-
sible recurrence. No matter how gently the clinician presents the
facts, he is acutely aware that the patient's hopes for a continuing cancer-free future will be dashed all to hell, his emotional
equilibrium knocked for a loop, and his life suspended, once again,
in medical limbo until the cancer is found and (hopefully) de-
stroyed.*

    *It is always difficult to deliver bad news, harder still when
the patient is a friend.*

Driving home, I thought about how to break the news to Rose.
There was no easy way, and the answer had to be swift. Any
hedging could only worsen the implications of the situation. But
maybe the news could be softened somehow, lightened up a touch
so as to put a good face on it, make it sound less dire. If I treated it
lightly, perhaps that would minimize the shock of hearing about it. I
didn't believe myself for a minute, but continued to pursue the way
to spin this issue..

    "Hi, honey—how'd it go?" Rose asks, as I knew she would.
    "Well, it looks like we may add another chapter to the book,"
I answer with as much nonchalance as I can muster.
    "You worked on that line all the way home, didn't you?"
    "Yeah, I did."
    "Too bad it didn't work. What did Tom say?"
    I tell her about the elevated PSA and what it might portend;
also about the possibility that there was a lab or biological anomaly,
and that another blood test was in progress as we spoke.
    "When will we know the results?"

"Couple of days."

"What if wasn't a lab variation?"

"More tests, radiation, maybe hormones, whatever it takes to get rid of it." I didn't have to paint her a picture. There was nothing further to say, and so we each retreated to our own private hells, the thrill of becoming grandparents buried beneath the cloud of this new state of affairs.

That night, I came down with all the flu-like symptoms Nyquil promises to alleviate. My immune system was obviously traumatized by the depressing news, and let the virus gain enough of a hold to take me down. I foresaw at least a week of upper respiratory misery and general malaise. On the positive side, my head was reeling so badly from an elevated temperature, I couldn't think about the latest forebodings. For two days, barely able to get out of bed, my thoughts consisted only of whether I was struggling to get to the bathroom to vomit, or to have another bout of diarrhea. For two merciful, days, I didn't think about prostate cancer. For two days, Rose looked sicker than I felt.

On the third day, the phone rang before the business day even started. It was Tom, who excitedly told me he had just received my lab report and it was less than zero point two, that the earlier one was, indeed, a lab anomaly.

"You mean I don't have to see you in two weeks?"

"The next time I want to see you, except for dinner, is in six months."

Our joy could have melted the phone lines. And as if I had gulped some magical elixir, my flu symptoms lifted. Obviously, the good, great, wonderful, miraculous, fabulous news got the thumb-sucking, sulking old immune system up and running in what may be record time. The fact that my first grandson decided to join the world that day no doubt hastened the recovery to some degree as well. The day was so bright it made my eyes tear.

Daybook Entry, 10/24/97

<u>Patient:</u> Bert Gottlieb
<u>PSA:</u> 0.2 Ng/Ml
<u>Call to patient:</u> As soon as I received the lab report, I phoned Bert with the results. He couldn't have been happier, nor could I. And since we had both just become grandfathers (my third), there was even more good news to celebrate.
<u>Management:</u> Return in 6 months. PSA prior to visit.

This is the end of the book, but not the end of the story. Twice a year, I have to put my life on hold until I know my PSA is okay and I can breathe again.

The high I get from hearing an almost immeasurable PSA number keeps me buoyant for months, affirming to me (though contrary to clinical statistics, I know) that I'm one of the lucky ones, one of the cured. Talk to me in five years. Maybe then I'll be able to say, "I used to have prostate cancer."

* * *

RECOMMENDED READING

The Men's Club was never intended to cover all the ground necessary to a complete understanding of every aspect of prostate cancer. To that end, the authors recommend the following books, which examine the subject from many other important points of view. There is much to be learned from them including, to a greater or lesser degree, important information about resources and support groups available to anyone interested in up-to-the-minute prostate cancer facts.

Prostate Cancer: A Family Guide to Diagnosis, Treatment & Survival
Sheldon Marks, M.D.
Fisher Books, 1995

Prostate Cancer: A Guide for Women and the Men They Love
Barbara Wainrib with Sandra Haber
Dell Trade Paperback, 1996

Prostate Cancer: What Every Man— and His Family— Needs to Know
David Bostwick M.D., Gregory T. MacLennan M.D., and Thayne R. Larson M.D.
Villard, 1996

Prostate Disease
W. Scott McDougal, MD., with P.J. Skerrett
Times Book, division of Random House, 1996

The ABCs of Prostate Cancer
Joseph E., Oesterling, M.D., with Mark A. Mayad
Madison Books, 1997

The Patient's Guide to Prostate Cancer
Marc Garnick, M.D.
Plume Books, 1996

The Prostate: A Guide For Men and the Women Who Love Them
Patrick Walsh, M.D., with Janet Farrar Worthington
Warner Books, 1995

NOTES

NOTES

NOTES

Pathfinder Publishing of California
3600 Harbor Blvd, # 82
Oxnard, CA   93035
Telephone 805-984-7756   Fax: 805-985-3267
Please call for Pricing and Delivery Information for other Pathfinder
Publishing:Books :
Web Page: Pathfinderpublishing.com